DIAGNOSTIC PICTURE TESTS IN

OBS'

& GYNAECOLOGY

Hilary Joyce MBBS,MRACOG (Tutor/Registrar)
Janet F. Patrick BSc,MBChB,MRCOG (Tutor)
Geoffrey D. Reid MBBS,MRACOG (Lecturer)
Frank L. Wilcox MD,MRCOG (Lecturer)
Professor **Victor R. Tindall**
MD,MSc,FRCS,FRCOG
(Head of Department)
De⋯⋯⋯ ⋯ ⋯⋯⋯⋯⋯ and Gynaecology

Titles published in the Diagnostic Picture Tests in . . . series include:

Picture Tests in Human Anatomy
DPT in Cardiology
DPT in Clinical Medicine, Vol 1–4
DPT in Clinical Neurology
DPT in Dermatology
DPT in Ear, Nose and Throat
DPT in Embryology
DPT in Endocrinology
DPT in Gastroenterology
DPT in General Dentistry
DPT in General Medicine
DPT in General Surgery
DPT in Geriatric Medicine
DPT in Infectious Diseases
Differential Diagnosis in AIDS

400 Self Assessment Picture Tests in Clinical Medicine
DPT in Injury in Sport
DPT in Ophthalmology
DPT in Oral Medicine
DPT in Orthopaedics
DPT in Paediatrics, 2nd edn
DPT in Paediatric Dentistry
DPT in Respiratory Disease
DPT in Rheumatology
DPT in Urology
400 More Self Assessment Picture Tests in Clinical Medicine

Copyright © V.R.Tindall, 1987
Published in 1987 by Wolfe Medical Publications Ltd.
Printed by BPCC Hazell Books, Aylesbury, Bucks, England
ISBN 0 7234 0932 3
Reprinted 1994 by Wolfe Publishing, an imprint of Mosby–Year Book
Europe Limited

For full details of all Mosby–Year Book Europe Limited titles please write to Mosby–Year Book Europe Limited, Lynton House, 7–12 Tavistock Square, London WC1H 9LB, England.

Preface

When it was suggested that a book of this type was required for undergraduates and postgraduates, we were already experimenting with this method of assessing undergraduate clinical experience with tape/slide examinations. Our experience was favourable and we believed that when presented in book format, it would provide an additional and valuable teaching aid.

The book is a team effort from the Department of Obstetrics, each of whom is heavily involved in teaching undergraduate and postgraduate students and has in the past suffered at the hands of examiners. The illustrations, questions and answers, therefore, have been subject to much criticism in the process of generation.

Our format is asking four questions for each illustration. Commonly, one question asks for the possible diagnosis but the others may or may not be related directly to the illustration. This has allowed us to pose questions appropriate for undergraduates or postgraduates, although both groups will benefit from the easier questions because it is often the error of omission which fails a candidate in an examination, missing the obvious and simple fact, not the difficult or abstruse one.

We have not by any means covered the whole field of obstetrics and gynaecology and did not intend to do so because we regard this book as a learning aid. We hope that readers will look at any picture in a text book or colour atlas in a different manner in future and will ask themselves questions about what they see rather than just accepting what is written. If so, we have achieved our aim, namely to help and stimulate our undergraduate and postgraduate readers, whether or not they are taking examinations.

Acknowledgements

We wish to thank the Department of Medical Illustration at the Manchester Royal Infirmary for their assistance with the duplication of the slides which are included, as well as those additional ones which were originally considered for inclusion. The collection could never have been obtained without the generous co-operation of many friends and colleagues: Dr P Buck, Dr C H Buckley, Dr R W Burslem, Dr P Donnai, Professor C P Douglas, Dr L Goss, Dr V Jones, Dr B A Lieberman, Dr J Richens, Dr S Rimmer, Dr D W Warrell and the late Mrs K Lamb.

We are particularly grateful to Miss Jane Holt for her typing, and co-ordination of the five authors, for out of the chaos generated, this book finally emerged. Therefore, we would like to dedicate the book to her as a token of our appreciation for making it possible, despite our heavy clinical duties.

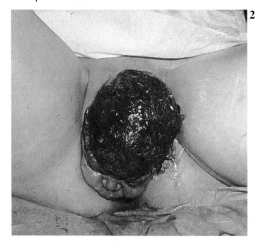

1 (a) What is the surgical procedure being performed?
(b) What are the potential benefits of the procedure? — *Mother + feta*
(c) What are the potential hazards of the procedure?
(d) What are the alternative incisions?

2 (a) Which complication of delivery may occur at this stage?
(b) In which patients is this most likely to occur?
(c) Which fetal injury may result from excessive traction?
(d) What was the presentation?

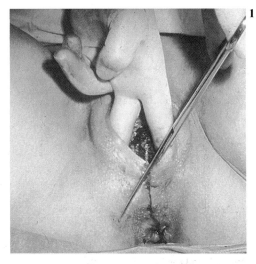

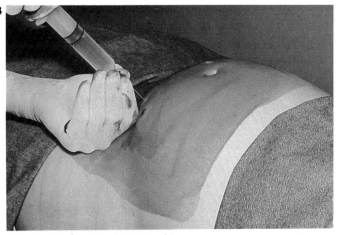

3 The patient is Rh negative.
(a) What diagnostic procedure is being performed and why?
(b) What other procedures may be helpful in the management of this pregnancy?
(c) What are the other diagnostic applications of this procedure?
(d) Name some common complications of the procedure

4 A woman presented with hyperemis gravidarum and bleeding per vaginum. The uterus was larger than expected for her dates and she passed the tissue shown.
(a) What is the diagnosis?
(b) How may the patient present?
(c) What is the usual chromosome pattern?
(d) What biochemical measurements should be carried out?

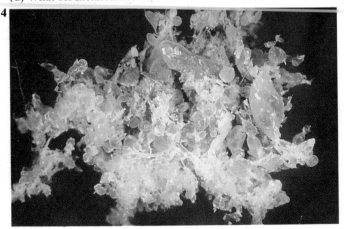

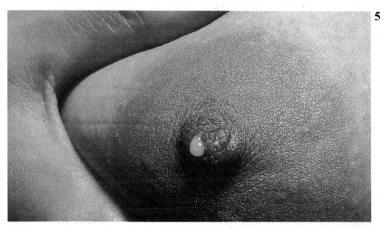

5 The patient complained of galactorrhoea, infrequent periods and infertility.
(a) Which hormone assay would help in making a diagnosis?
(b) If the hormone level were elevated, what other investigations should be arranged?
(c) If an abnormality were found, what medical treatment might be indicated?
(d) If an abnormality were found, what surgical treatment is occasionally required?

6 (a) What is the most likely diagnosis in this woman from Papua New Guinea?
(b) What is it likely to be mistaken for?
(c) How would the diagnosis of the two conditions be confirmed?
(d) Is elephantiasis a recognised complication of this condition?

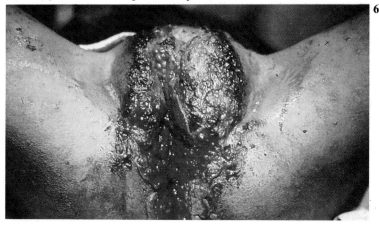

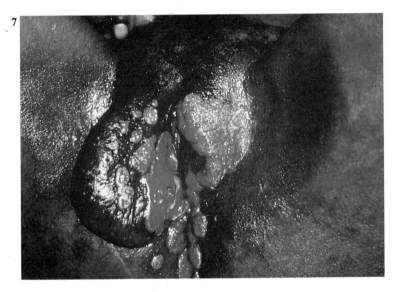

7

7,8 Smears from the lesions (**7**) showed the intracellular inclusions in **8**.
(a) What are the inclusions called?
(b) What is the organism?
(c) Which tissues are predominantly affected?
(d) Which are the most common extra genital sites for this infection?

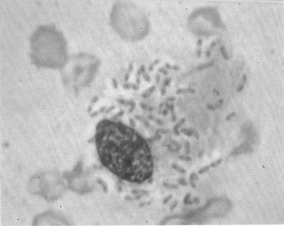

8

9 Lymphoedema and elephantiasis of the vulva.

(a) After surgical removal of this large tumour is there likely to be a recurrence?

(b) Give 3 main causes of obstruction to the lymphatics of the vulva.

(c) Give 3 causes of swellings of the vulva which are not associated with lymphatic obstruction.

(d) Is the ulcerated area of this tumour likely to be painful or painless?

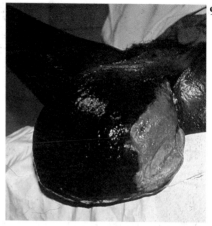

10 (a) What is the immediate reaction as to the nature of this vulval tumour?

(b) How would the diagnosis be established?

(c) If malignant, what is the survival related to?

(d) Which group of melanomas are associated with virtually a 100 per cent, 5-year survival?

11 This pelvic mass was removed at laparotomy.

(a) What is it?

(b) List the degenerative changes that may occur.

(c) What are the likely symptoms?

(d) What might be the age of this patient?

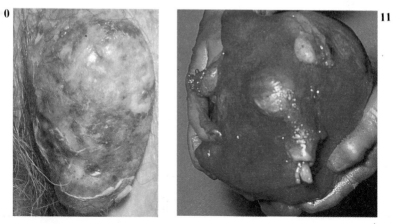

12

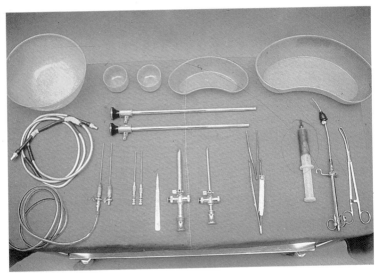

12 (a) Name the instruments on this operation tray.
(b) What is the alternative type of trochar?
(c) What gas might be used during the use of these instruments?
(d) What additional equipment would be required for a sterilisation operation?

13 (a) What is illustrated?
(b) With what symptoms may the patient have presented?
(c) What are the most common findings on pelvic examination?
(d) What investigations may help to make the diagnosis?

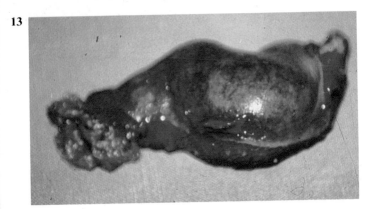

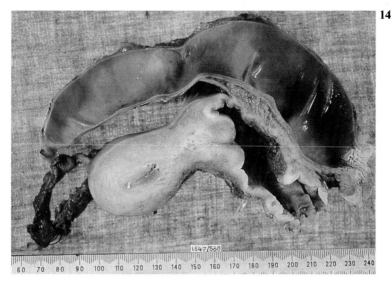

14 (a) What viscera are shown?
(b) What surgical procedure has been performed? *Exenteration*
(c) Why was this surgical resection performed?
(d) To which group of lymph nodes may this disseminate?

15 (a) What is this structure?
(b) What hormones influence its development and where are they produced?
(c) What is likely to happen to it?
(d) How many chromosomes are in the oocyte? *not chromatids*

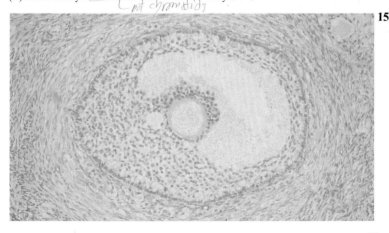

16

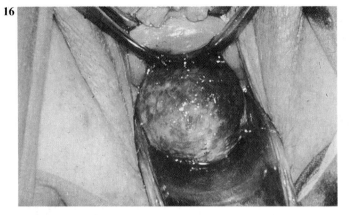

16 This patient was found to have a mass extruding through the cervix.
(a) What is the most likely diagnosis?
(b) List two other possible causes.
(c) What is the management of this condition in a patient wishing to conserve her fertility?
(d) If the subsequent pathology after conservative surgery were malignant what would be the course of action?

Caroncle   ?

17

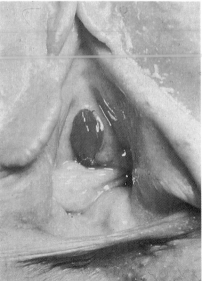

Urethral opening 6 Brisht red polypoid growth

17 (a) What is shown?
(b) What is the differential diagnosis?
(c) What are the histological types of this abnormality?
(d) If malignant, what is the treatment of choice?

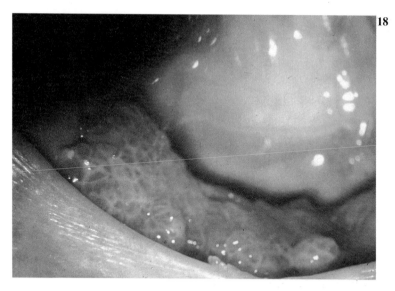

18,19 (a) What is the condition illustrated?
(b) What specific information should be sought in history-taking?
(c) In what percentage of 'at risk' patients is this abnormality present?
(d) What is the incidence of malignant change?

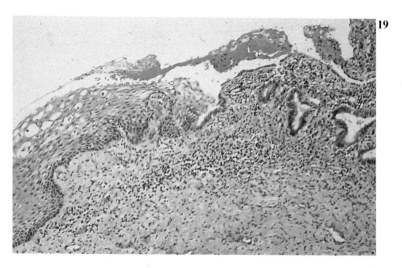

20

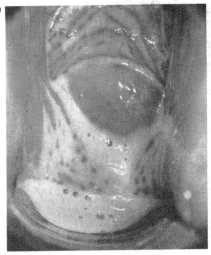

20 This patient was admitted with an acute salpingitis.
(a) What is the likely cause?
(b) How would the cause be determined?
(c) What blood tests are appropriate?
(d) What treatment should be given while waiting for the results?

21 (a) What surgical procedure is being carried out?
(b) What is the rationale for the operation?
(c) What is the potential disadvantage of the operation?
(d) What medical treatment(s) should be considered for a patient wishing to conceive?

21

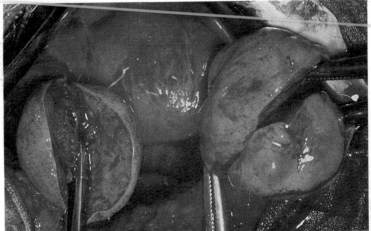

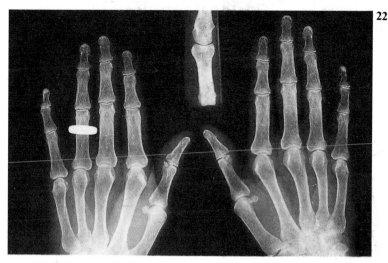

22 An X-ray of the hands of a woman aged 60 years and, for comparison, an X-ray of a 30-year-old woman's finger is shown in the centre.
(a) What is the diagnosis?
(b) What is the aetiology? bone resorption > bone mineralization = ↓ bone mass density
(c) What is the effect of exercise on this process? improve
(d) What is the effect of excessive smoking? worsens condition

23 This photograph was taken at laparotomy.
(a) What is visible on the right side of the uterus?
(b) What type is it?
(c) Where could it have come from?
(d) Is there anything to be stressed in any future pregnancy?

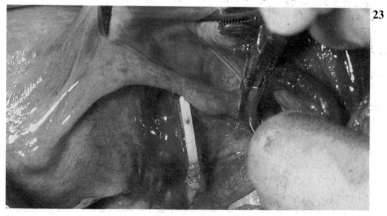

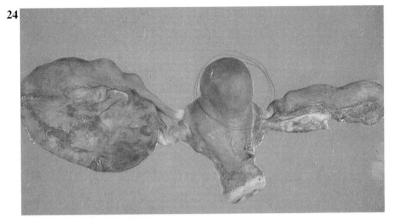

24 Carcinoma of the Fallopian tube.
(a) Is there evidence of secondary spread?
(b) Is this rare tumour more common before or after the menopause?
(c) What is the usual histological pattern?
(d) Why is the prognosis poor?

25 (a) What is the nature of these uterine tumours?
(b) Where has the large tumour on the left been located?
(c) Is any particular structure at risk?
(d) What is likely to have been the presenting symptom?

25

26 (a) What is this condition called when it arises in pregnancy?
(b) What two characteristic features are shown?
(c) What is the aetiology?
(d) Does it recur?

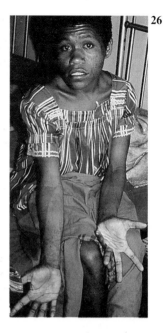

27 This is a rare dermatological disease peculiar to pregnancy.
(a) What is it called?
(b) What is the usual presenting symptom?
(c) What is the treatment of choice?
(d) Can the fetus be similarly affected?

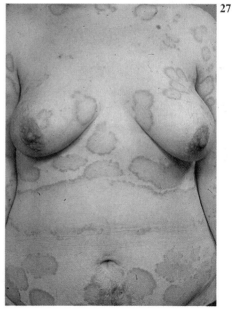

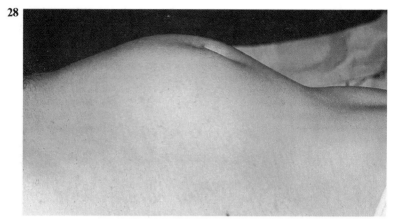

28,29 (a) What is this condition?
(b) How is it likely to present?
(c) What is the cause?
(d) How is it treated?

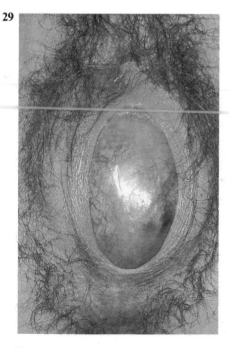

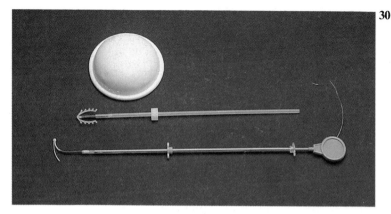

30 (a) Name these three contraceptive devices.
(b) What is the failure rate of the barrier device?
(c) What is the failure rate of the non-barrier devices?
(d) What are the risks of the non-barrier devices?

31 (a) Describe the features of this X-ray.
(b) What may occur during breech delivery to suggest this diagnosis?
(c) What further complications will occur during delivery?
(d) What procedure should be performed in these circumstances?

Able to fertili
since bones
are not
fused)

Huge skull! —

31

Normal

LO Cephalic

OA @ delivery

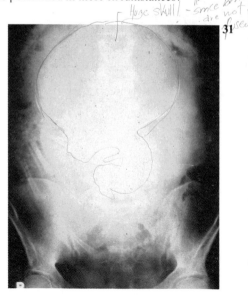

32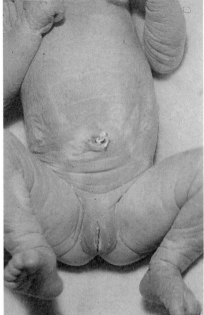

32 This baby was delivered following induction of labour at 295 days after the last menstrual period.
(a) What was the likely indication for induction of labour?
(b) What are the features of an infant with this condition?
(c) What would be the obstetric risks of having allowed the pregnancy to continue?
(d) What are the features of the placenta in this type of case?

33 (a) Describe the abnormal features on this cardiotocograph recording.
(b) What action is necessary?
(c) Is there any necessity to discontinue the Syntocinon infusion?
(d) Are the contractions excessive in frequency or strength?

33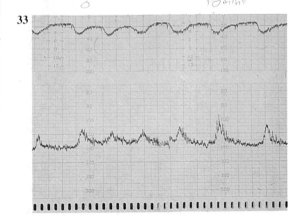

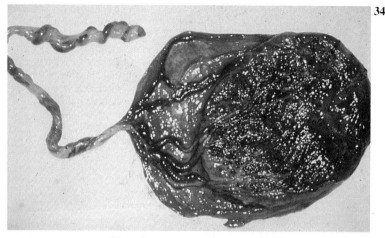

34 (a) Name the condition shown.
(b) What is the most likely complication? *Vasa praevia*
(c) How would this complication be recognised clinically?
(d) Is there any blood test that may be of use with this complication?

35 Although an intravenous pyelogram (IVP) is rarely indicated in pregnancy one had been performed in this patient. The X-ray shown was taken 40 minutes after injection of the contrast material.
(a) What renal abnormality is demonstrated?
(b) What ureteric abnormality is seen on the left?
(c) Is the fetal skeleton normal?
(d) From this IVP, is there enough justification to suggest that the baby should be delivered early?

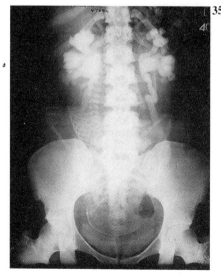

36

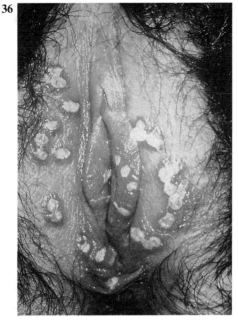

36 (a) What is the most likely diagnosis?
(b) How is the patient likely to present?
(c) What investigations should be performed?
(d) What is the natural history?

37

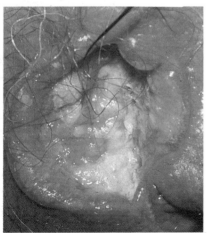

37 A 55-year-old woman recently developed a vulval lesion. She complained of weight loss, tiredness and breathlessness. She had an enlarged spleen.
(a) What is the lesion shown and what common laboratory investigations may support the diagnosis pre-operatively?
(b) What other procedure would confirm the diagnosis?
(c) What is the treatment for this lesion?
(d) What chromosome abnormality is associated?

38 This is elephantiasis due to filariasis.

(a) Is the oedema usually asymmetrical?

(b) What other feature is present?

(c) If the inguinal lymph nodes are involved, are they likely to harbour the parasite?

(d) On histological examination of the lymph nodes, if no trace of a dead worm is found, what other condition gives a similar histological appearance?

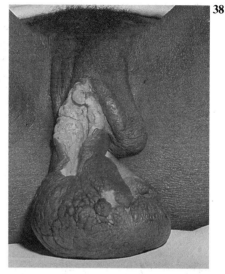

39,40 (a) What is the diagnosis?

(b) What is the treatment?

(c) How would bleeding be prevented?

(d) What is the small ulcer likely to be due to?

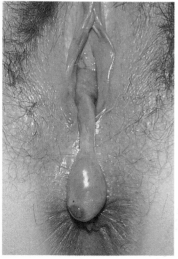

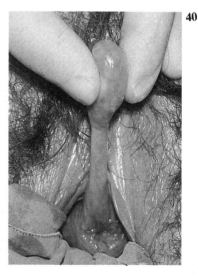

41

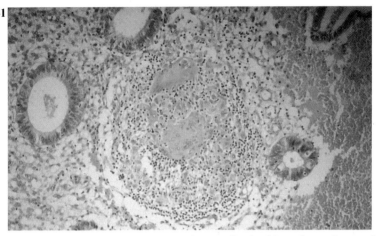

41 (a) What is responsible for the abnormality in this endometrium and how would it be confirmed?
(b) What is the likely presenting complaint?
(c) How does it spread?
(d) What is the treatment?

42 This was removed from an 18-year-old woman ten days after the spontaneous expulsion of a missed abortion; she was admitted to Casualty Department ten hours prior to its removal.
(a) She presented with cardiopulmonary collapse. What were the presenting symptoms?
(b) What is it?
(c) Following recovery, what method of contraceptive would be advisable?
(d) What treatment should be recommended in her next pregnancy? What possible complications might arise in it?

42

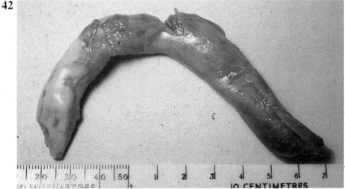

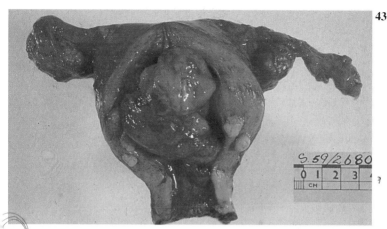

S 59/2680

43 This is a mixed Mullerian tumour.
(a) In what age group do these tumours usually present?
(b) What are the common symptoms?
(c) Is this one of the tumours in which fragments of necrotic tumour may be passed per vagina?
(d) From what tissue do these tumours arise?

44 The graph represents the incidence of carcinoma of the cervix in the United Kingdom between 1968 and 1979.
(a) What is the major difference between 1968 and 1979?
(b) What is the significance of this difference?
(c) Are there any possible explanations for this change?
(d) Is there evidence from the graph that cervical cytology screening has helped?

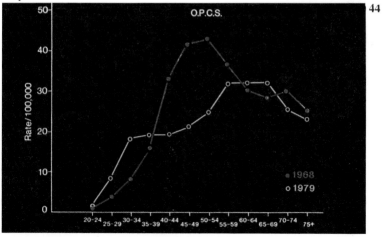

45

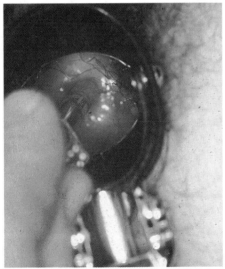

45 (a) How may such a giant ovarian cyst be differentiated from ascites?
(b) Which investigation would be most helpful pre-operatively?
(c) Was this cyst malignant or benign?
(d) If malignant, how should it be treated?

46

46 (a) What procedure is being performed?
(b) What are the features of ovulatory mucus?
(c) In what ways may cervical mucus contribute to infertility?
(d) What tests may be useful?

47 (a) What is the likely diagnosis?
(b) What is the aetiology?
(c) Do they cause symptoms?
(d) What is the treatment?

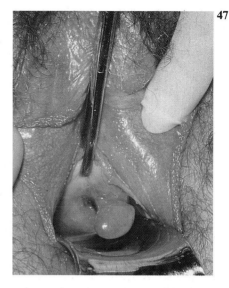

48 (a) Is this tumour more likely to be benign or malignant?
(b) If malignant, primary or secondary?
(c) What is the most likely cell type of this tumour?
(d) What is the prognosis?

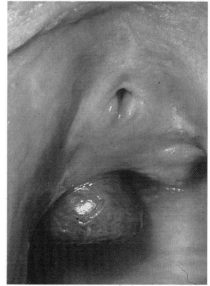

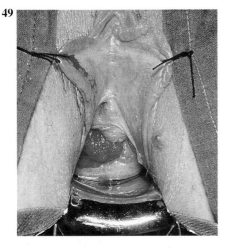

49,50 This patient is constantly wet.
(a) What is the diagnosis?
(b) What obstetric complication is a likely cause?
(c) Name two infective causes.
(d) What is the best treatment?

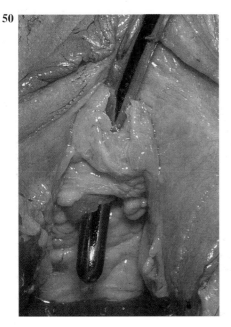

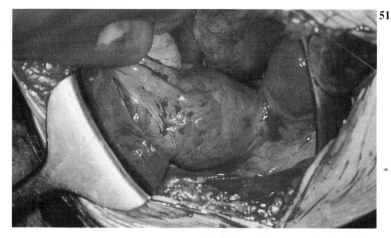

51 This woman was undergoing hysterectomy for menorrhagia.
(a) What abnormality is present?
(b) What pre-operative investigation should have been performed?
(c) What particular hazard should the surgeon be aware of?
(d) What operation might have been performed to correct the abnormality?

52 The incidence of choriocarcinoma in the omentum varies from country to country.
(a) In which parts of the world is it highest?
(b) In what proportion of cases would it follow a hydatidiform mole?
(c) Is the age incidence more common in women over or under 35 years?
(d) What is the present-day cure rate?

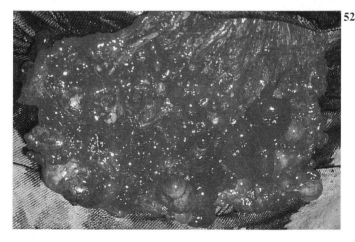

53

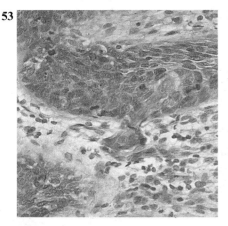

53 (a) What disease is shown in this biopsy taken from the vulva?

(b) What epidemiological change has occurred with this disease over recent years?

(c) Which other disease is frequently present in patients with this condition?

(d) Which factors influence the prognosis?

54

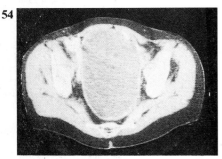

54 (a) Describe what is seen in this CAT scan.

(b) What is the diagnosis?

(c) What more usual imaging technique may be used?

(d) What is the chance of malignancy?

55 This is a trace produced during multi-channel cystometry.

(a) What are the three traces measuring?

(b) Is the capacity (280 ml) normal?

(c) Is the first desire (about 20 ml) normal?

(d) Is any detrusor activity demonstrated?

55

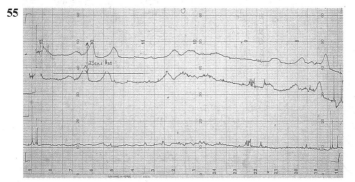

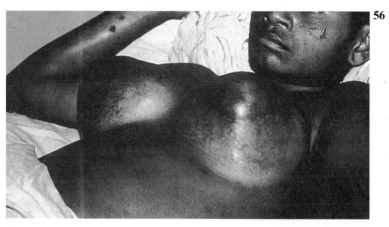

56 (a) What is illustrated?
(b) When does this usually occur?
(c) What may ensue?
(d) What drugs might give relief?

57 (a) What lesion is present?
(b) Is it likely to result from infection or malignancy?
(c) Is it likely to produce Horner's syndrome?
(d) Which gynaecological lesions may produce this?

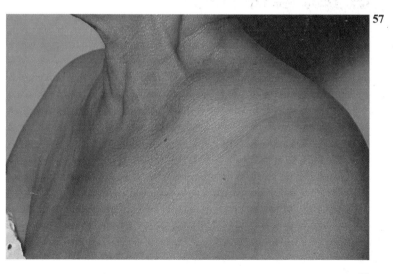

58

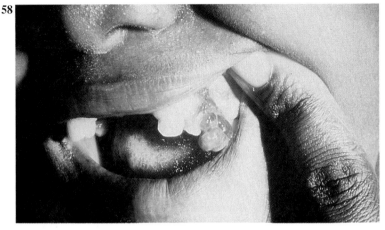

58 (a) What is the likely diagnosis?
(b) What complication might occur?
(c) What is the usual sequela?
(d) Is the condition characteristically associated with tooth decay?

59 The partner of this patient had a urethral discharge.
(a) What is the likely diagnosis?
(b) What other joints may be affected?
(c) How may the diagnosis be confirmed?
(d) What other tests should be done?

59

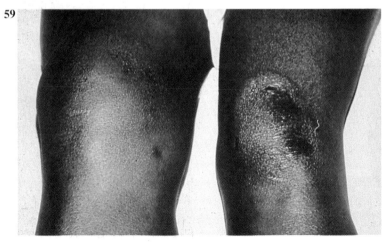

60 (a) What is the obvious diagnosis?
(b) What are the classical features?
(c) What other associated abnormalites are recognised?
(d) Are there any variants of this condition?

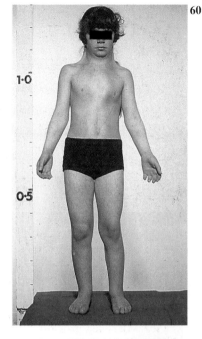

61 (a) From which disease does the mother of this baby suffer?
(b) What treatment should the mother have throughout the antenatal period in another pregnancy?
(c) What are the risks to the neonate?
(d) Is it an hereditary disorder?

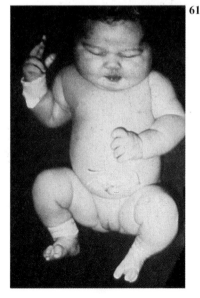

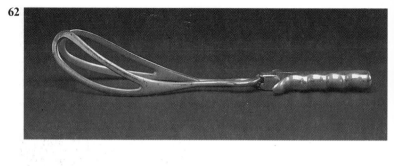

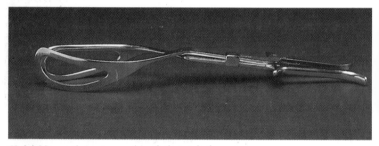

62 (a) Name these two pairs of obstetric forceps.
(b) What are the principal differences?
(c) For what use are the lower forceps suited?
(d) For what purpose were the lower forceps originally intended?

63 (a) What abnormalities of the limbs are shown in this X-ray?
(b) What abnormalities of the head and trunk are shown?
(c) What is this condition?
(d) What particular labour complications may be anticipated?

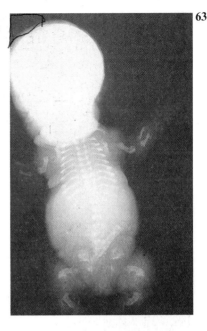

64 (a) What does this placenta demonstrate?
(b) Is there any recognised complication prior to the onset of labour?
(c) How may this complication present in labour?
(d) What postpartum problem may arise?

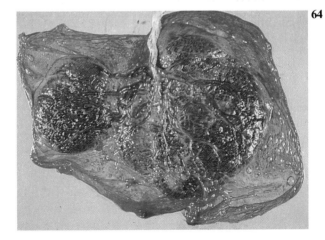

65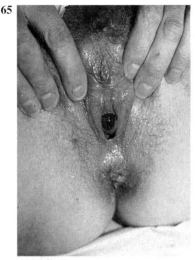

65 (a) What are the possible causes of this painful urethral swelling?

(b) How would the diagnosis be established?

(c) If this had been present for a long time and then suddenly became painful, what is a possible cause?

(d) Are there likely to be any associated gynaecological lesions?

66,67 An unusual lesion of the clitoris which is caused by *Entamoeba histolytica* is shown in **66**. The organisms seen on scrapings from the lesion are shown in **67**.

(a) In countries where intestinal infection with this is endemic, is anogenital infection a well recognised complication?

(b) Is this type of lesion likely to be accompanied by intestinal symptoms?

(c) Is the lesion usually painful or painless?

(d) Would the finding of granulation tissue formation in these lesions be expected?

66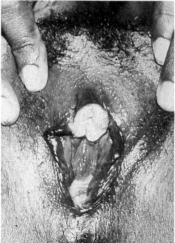

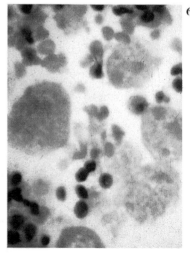

68 (a) What type of connective tissue neoplasm might this be?
(b) Which particular neoplasms are likely to reach the size of this tumour?
(c) Is ulceration common?
(d) Are the lymph nodes likely to be enlarged?

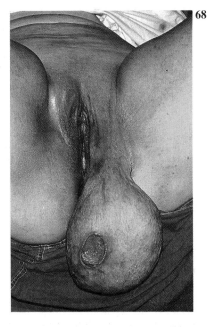

69 (a) What is the diagnosis and can it be made with certainty?
(b) What are the chances of a successful cure?
(c) If the uterus had been removed abdominally previously, is the success rate as good?
(d) Would coital function have to be sacrificed?

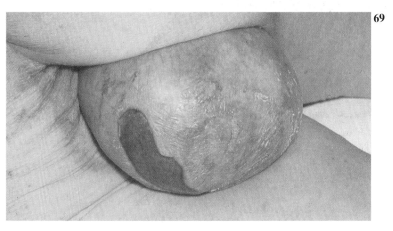

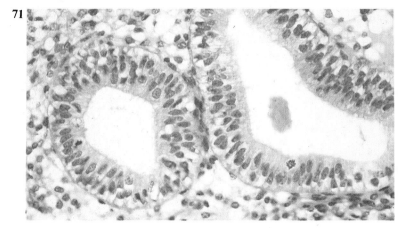

70 (a) What lesions are shown in this part of a uterus?
(b) What age is this patient likely to be?
(c) What were the probable presenting complaints?
(d) What would be the principal clinical finding?

71 (a) What is shown?
(b) How might it have been obtained?
(c) When was it obtained?
(d) What is its significance?

72 This placenta was morbidly adherent and hysterectomy was required for its removal.
(a) What is the recommended treatment in the condition of placenta acreta where the placenta cannot be separated and there is no bleeding?
(b) If this treatment is followed, will laceration occur?
(c) How long is it before menstruation commonly returns?
(d) What other examples of abnormal adherence of the placenta are there?

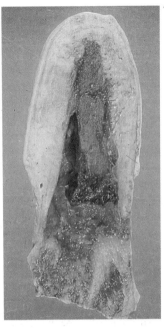

73 (a) What uterine abnormality is displayed?
(b) Is there any additional feature present?
(c) What obstetrical malpresentation may have been found in this patient?
(d) What complications are commonly associated with this abnormality in labour?

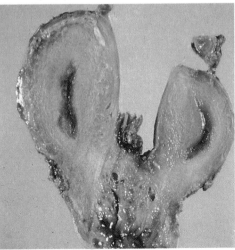

74

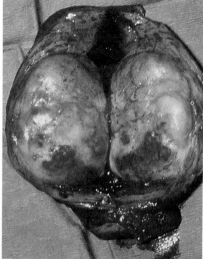

74 The uterus was removed because it was felt that the patient's anaemia was due to menorrhagia associated with a fibroid uterus.

(a) The histology was reported as showing a sarcomatous lesion. What should be done?

(b) Should the diagnosis have been expected from the macroscopic appearance?

(c) What is the chance of malignant change occurring in a fibroid?

(d) Would the possiblity of malignant change alter the management of leiomyomata?

75

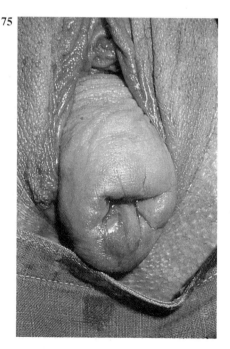

75 (a) With what symptoms would this patient present?

(b) What factors contribute to this condition?

(c) What is the treatment of choice?

(d) What is an alternative treatment?

76 The patient is 22 weeks pregnant.

(a) What abnormality is seen?

(b) She has no pain; what is the diagnosis?

(c) What are the possible causes?

(d) What is the treatment?

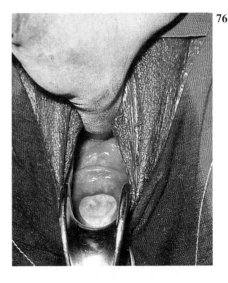

77 An early carcinoma of the cervix is shown.

(a) From the size of the vaginal cervix, is the patient more likely to have been aged 30 years or 50 years?

(b) What investigation is necessary before treatment is started?

(c) Would colposcopy be helpful?

(d) What type of carcinoma is it likely to be?

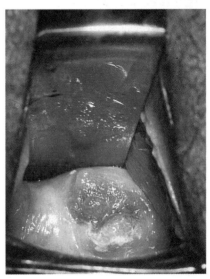

78

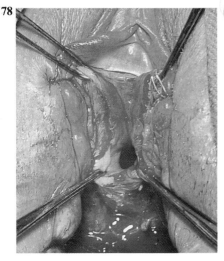

78 A fibrosed, thickened urethra opened longitudinally is shown. Note the dilated internal meatus. The patient has had a long history of stress incontinence.

(a) What is the likely cause of the urethral fibrosis?

(b) She is completely incontinent now. Why?

(c) What can be done to relieve her incontinence?

(d) What types of incontinence are there?

79 (a) What is shown in this picture?

(b) What other abnormality may be associated with this condition?

(c) The patient complained of dysmenorrhoea. How should she be treated? ① irona ② Transaemic acid

(d) What obstetrical complications may be encountered?
Uterine abnormalities: ↑ Premature labour, abortion & malpresentation

79

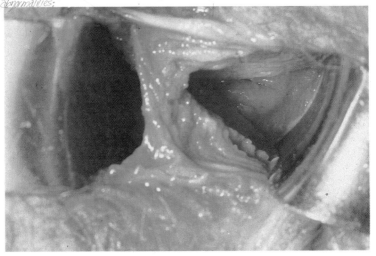

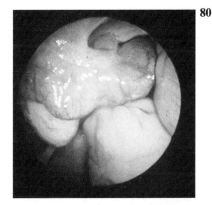

80 (a) What structures are visible in this laparoscopic view of the pelvis?
(b) What investigation is being carried out and for what purpose?
(c) Are the appearances within normal limits?
(d) What are the risks of this operation? Perforation
· Infection
· Haemorrhage
· Embolic accident

81 (a) What complication has occurred with this ovarian cyst?
(b) Is it possible to be surgically conservative?
(c) What other complications may occur?
(d) What is likely to be the presenting symptom of all these complications?

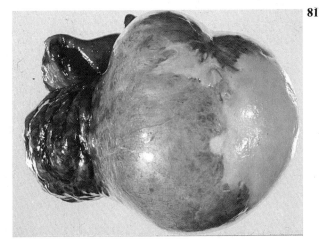

82

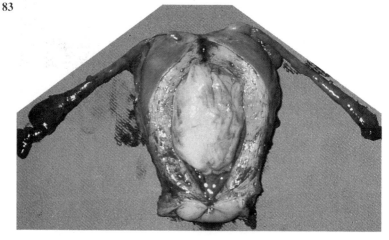

82 (a) What abnormality is present in this lateral skull X-ray?
(b) What hormone level is likely to be raised?
(c) What symptoms may the patient have?
(d) What other investigations should be made?

83 (a) What might this patient have complained of?
(b) To which age group does she belong?
(c) What is the diagnosis?
(d) Would this contain functional endometrium?

83

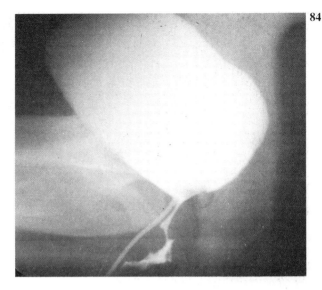

84 (a) What does this X-ray show?
(b) Name some possible causes.
(c) How may the symptoms vary, depending upon the site of the lesion?
(d) Is the patient likely to suffer from recurrent cystitis?

85 (a) Describe the features shown that would make one suspect pregnancy.
(b) Name another cause of this condition.
(c) What other features of the skin would be expected?
(d) Is it a permanent feature?

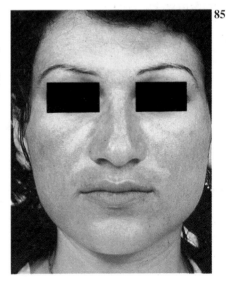

86

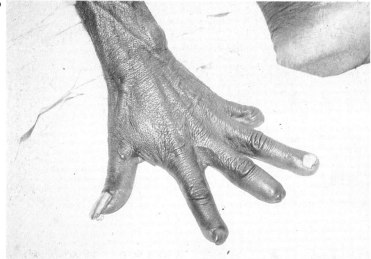

86 (a) Have these deformities any relevance to a patient's obstetric history?
(b) Can one estimate how many relatives have died?
(c) Suggest any other ritual procedure in women that may be carried out and what is a recognised complication of it?

87

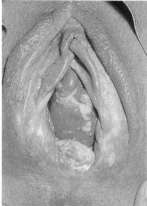

87 This 60-year-old patient presented with pruritus vulvae.
(a) What is the most likely infection and its treatment?
(b) What are the recognised predispositions to this type of infection?
(c) What other abnormal feature is seen?
(d) What treatment may be indicated for each of these abnormalities?

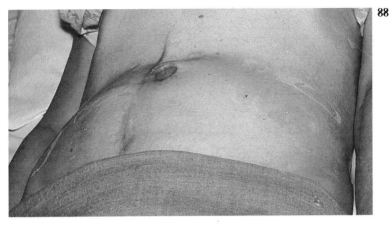

88,89 The patient in **88** had an ovarian carcinoma. The nodule (**89**) was removed 12 months later.
(a) What is the nodule?
(b) What are the likely causes of further lumps at this site?
(c) What is the mode of spread to this site?
(d) What sites are more usually involved?

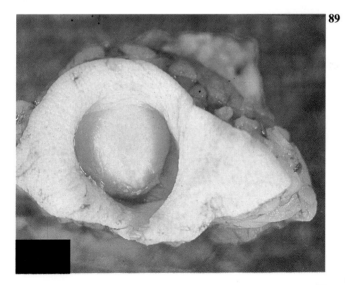

90

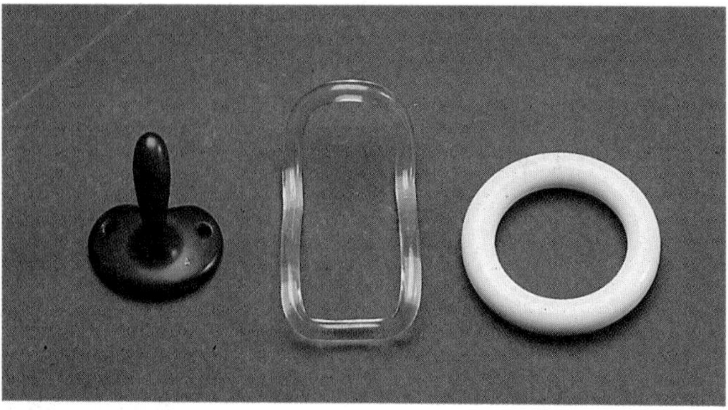

90 (a) Name these three devices.
(b) What is their intended use?
(c) What is a risk of their long-term use?
(d) How may this be minimised?

91 (a) What is the usual aetiology of liver palm noted in pregnancy?
(b) What other lesions may be present?
(c) It also may be noted in a patient who has a high intake of alcohol. If so, is the fetus likely to be affected in any way?
(d) What are the most sensitive indices of excessive alcohol consumption (more than 80 g/day) in pregnancy?

91

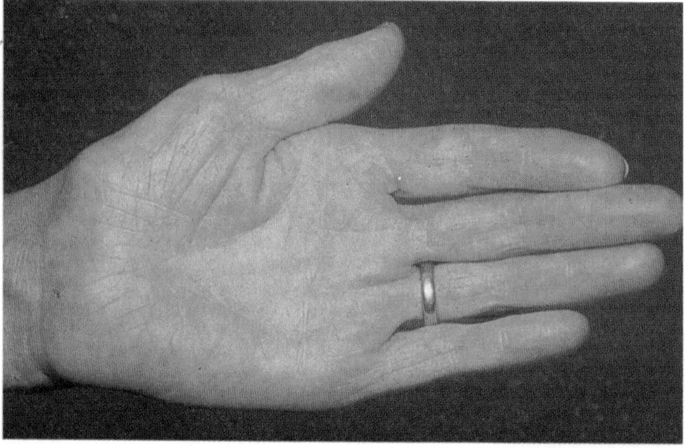

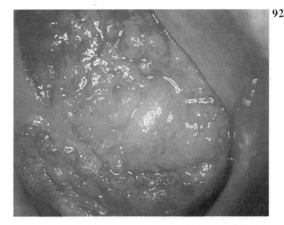

92 When this 25-year-old patient was 20 weeks pregnant she complained of slight blood loss vaginally and a speculum was passed.
(a) From the appearance, what could be the diagnosis?
(b) If the diagnosis were confirmed, what should be said to the patient?
(c) If the pregnancy is to continue, how should the care be managed?
(d) What is the long term prognosis?

93 (a) What are the abnormal features seen?
(b) What is the usual underlying biochemical abnormality?
(c) What is the phenotype, what are the gonads and what is the chromosomal pattern?
(d) How is it treated?

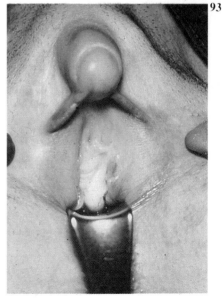

94

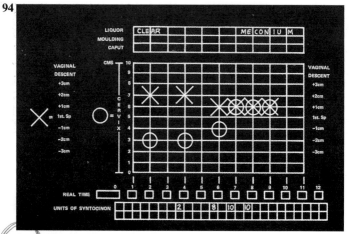

94 (a) What is the most important possible diagnosis?
(b) What features of the partogram may support this?
(c) What additional maternal signs may support the diagnosis?
(d) What additional information on the fetus may support the diagnosis?

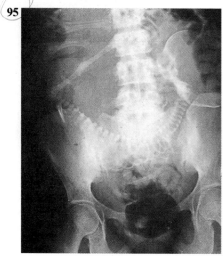

95 (a) Describe the lie of this fetus.
(b) What are the usual causes of this presentation?
(c) Is the fetus normal?
(d) What is the chance of an associated placenta praevia?

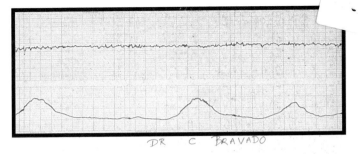

DR C BRAVADO

96 (a) What is the main abnormality seen in this cardiotocograph recording?
(b) What factors may cause this pattern?
(c) How does the significance of such a finding alter with gestation?
(d) Is this the typical response to normal uterine contractions?

97 This is an example of an ectopic gestation in which the rupture was from an unicornuate uterus.
(a) Does this type of catastrophe usually occur in the first or second trimester?
(b) Is there difficulty in establishing the diagnosis?
(c) Is it worth repairing the uterus after controlling the bleeding?
(d) Is it possible for the fetus to survive?

97

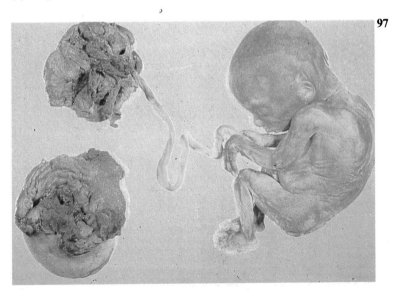

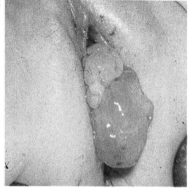

98 (a) What is the likely diagnosis in this 4-year-old girl?

(b) What are the most important characteristics in terms of prognosis?

(c) Has the treatment of this condition changed over the years?

(d) What are the most common signs?

99 (a) What is this lesion?
(b) What is the treatment?
(c) What is the incidence at this site?
(d) What is the prognosis?

100 The picture shows the lesions of chancroid.
(a) Is this sexually transmitted?
(b) What is the infecting organism?
(c) Are the lesions painful?
(d) What is the appropriate treatment?

99

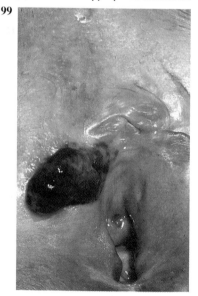

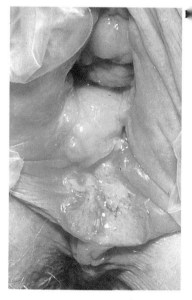

101,102 (a) What is the probable diagnosis?

(b) What is the patient's predominant symptom likely to be?

(c) At examination of the patient in the operating theatre, if the situation were assessed as in **102** what should be done?

(d) If corrected, would this be associated with loss of libido?

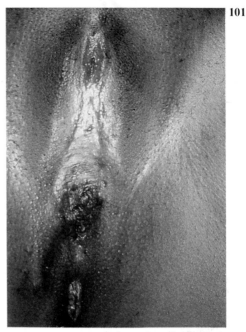

101

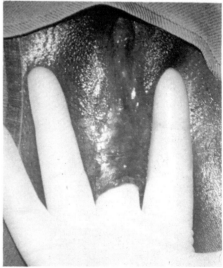

102

103 This woman had abnormal smears noted early in pregnancy.

(a) What procedure has been performed?

(b) Why may this have been carried out?

(c) What diagnostic procedures should have been performed prior to operation?

(d) What are the possible risks to a fetus?

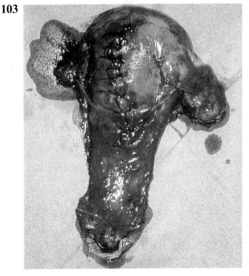

104 The patient attended for a routine smear at a Well Woman's Clinic. Cells from the smear are shown (magnification × 250).

(a) Are they normal or abnormal?

(b) Do they show mature, immature or both types of squamous cells?

(c) Is there evidence of squamous metaplasia; or of malignancy?

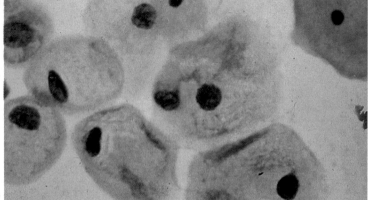

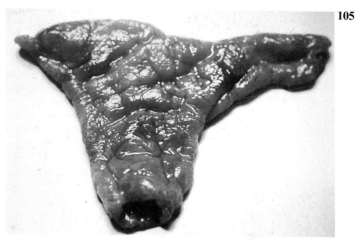

105 (a) What is this tissue which was passed *per vaginum*?
(b) With what potentially life-threatening condition may it be associated?
(c) With what may it be confused?
(d) In what other circumstances may it occur?

106 This specimen was removed from a patient with severe blood loss *per vaginum*.
(a) What is the likely diagnosis?
(b) Since both appendages were removed, in what probable age group is the patient?
(c) Apart from severe bleeding, how may the diagnosis be made?
(d) What is the estimated gestation of this patient?

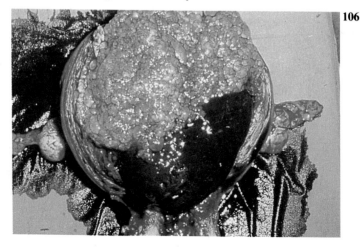

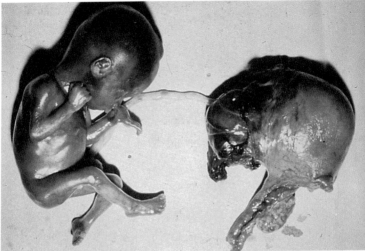

107 (a) What is the aetiology?
(b) It appears that the ovary has been removed. Is this justified in current practice?
(c) Name 3 other sites for this complication.
(d) What alternative outcome could have resulted from this pregnancy?

108 (a) Is this primary or secondary tuberculosis of the cervix?
(b) What are the usual macroscopic appearances of the cervix with this condition?

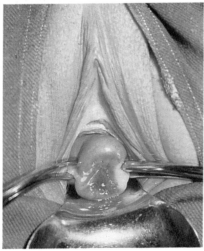

(c) What proportion of patients with tuberculosis of the Fallopian tubes are likely to have involvement of the cervix?
(d) Can it be sexually transmitted?

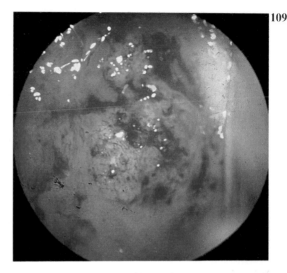

109 This is a colpophotograph with saline applied and magnification × 16. The vascular pattern can be seen in a lesion of the posterior lip of the cervix and there is also blood present.
(a) From where should a biopsy be taken? Assume that you are looking at a clockface and it is to be taken between two hours, eg 1–2, 2–3 etc.
(b) If the histology of a punch biopsy revealed microinvasion only, what should be done if the patient were aged 43 years?
(c) If the histology report revealed invasion squamous cell carcinoma and the patient were aged 33 years, what should be done?
(d) If the histology report revealed clear cell adenocarcinoma and the patient were aged 23 years, what should be done?

110 This is an uncommon infective ulcerative lesion of the cervix.
(a) It is rarely diagnosed and could resemble herpes infection of the cervix. Suggest a diagnosis.
(b) In its primary form approximately what proportion of patients have cervical involvement?
(c) Can it sometimes mimic a carcinoma?
(d) Apart from biopsy are there any specific tests to confirm the diagnosis and if the patient becomes pregnant, would the fetus be infected?

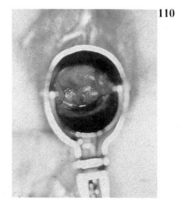

111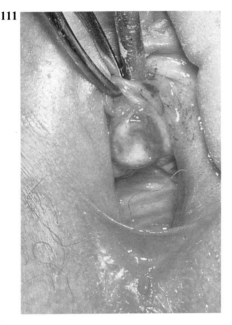

111 A vaginal lesion is shown.

(a) What is the most likely diagnosis in this patient who had a total abdominal hysterectomy and bilateral salpingo-oophorectomy 3 years previously?

(b) What is the treatment?

(c) What is the mode of spread?

(d) Could it have been avoided?

112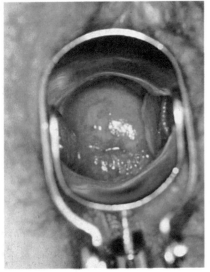

112 (a) What would a cervical smear be expected to reveal in this case?

(b) What is the diagnosis?

(c) What are the common agents responsible for this?

(d) What are the causes of infectious ulcers of the cervix?

113 (a) What structures are displayed in this picture?
(b) There is old longitudinal scarring of the anterior vaginal wall. What is the patient's complaint and why?
(c) How would this be repaired?
(d) What bladder drainage should be provided?

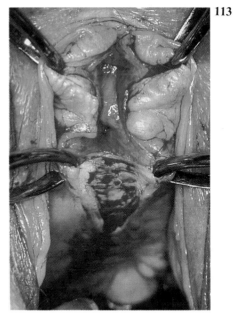

114 (a) In pregnancy, what are said to be the characteristic symptoms associated with this tumour (phaeochromocytoma)?
(b) Where does the tumour arise?
(c) Can they be malignant?
(d) How is the diagnosis confirmed or excluded?

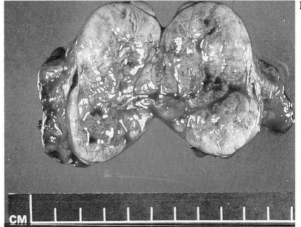

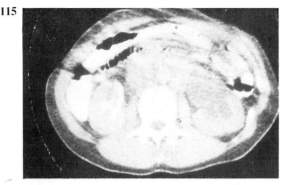

115 This shows a transverse abdominal CAT scan, at the level of the kidneys, taken during the investigation of a woman with carcinoma of the cervix.

(a) At what stage of cervical disease is this patient?

(b) In which patients with carcinoma of the cervix would CAT scans (if available) help in clinical management?

(c) What procedure can be performed in association with CAT scanning to confirm node involvement tumour?

(d) In which gynaecological tumours are CAT scans most likely to be helpful?

116 A benign ovarian cyst.

(a) What operative procedure should be carried out?

(b) Should the other ovary be biopsied?

(c) Would it be advisable to take peritoneal washings if there were no free fluid?

(d) Should the round ligaments be plicated?

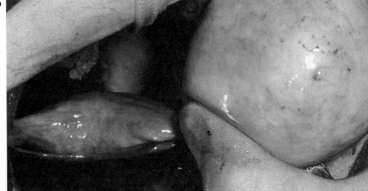

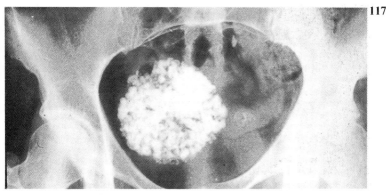

117 An X-ray of a 60-year-old patient who was involved in a road traffic accident.
(a) What are the abnormal features in this X-ray?
(b) What is the most likely diagnosis?
(c) What treatment is advisable?
(d) Suggest some possible complications.

118 This is a multi-channel cystometry trace.
(a) What filling media can be used for this investigation?
(b) How may these affect the results of the test?
(c) What other non-radiological studies of the lower renal tract may be useful in women with urinary symptoms?
(d) Does this picture show normal bladder pressure?

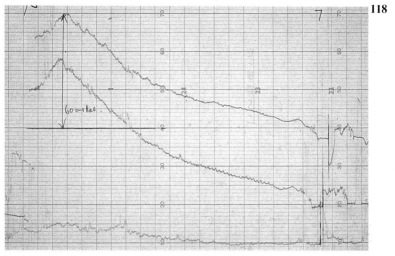

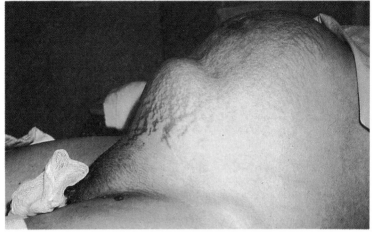

119 (a) What is the lower swelling caused by in this patient late in labour?
(b) How should it be dealt with?
(c) If this occurred in the antenatal period what would happen to the presenting part?
(d) Would this be compatible with a Bandl's ring?

120 (a) What abnormality is present in this postpartum patient?
(b) What is the likely cause?
(c) What related signs may also be present?
(d) What is the treatment?

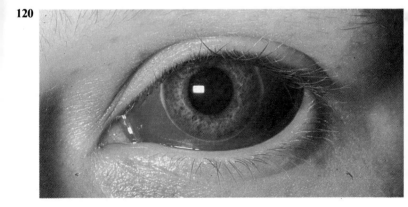

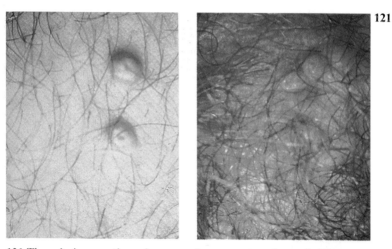

121 These lesions on the vulva were also present on the neck. They were found during the second pregnancy. Similar lesions were present during the first pregnancy.
(a) What is the likely diagnosis?
(b) What is their aetiology?
(c) If the lesions on the neck were pedunculated, how should they be treated?
(d) Where is another common site for these lesions?

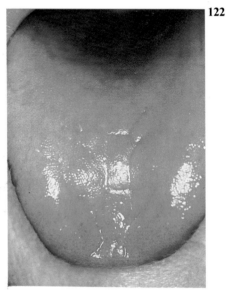

122 This patient complained of feeling tired and lethargic. She had a long history of menorrhagia.
(a) What is the probable cause?
(b) Where else would one look for clinical evidence to confirm the diagnosis?
(c) What would the blood film be expected to show?
(d) If the haemoglobin were less than 5 g/dl, how should the patient be treated?

123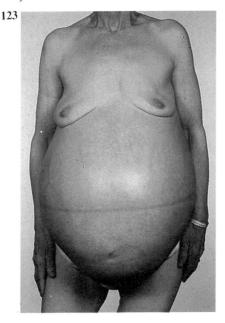

123 (a) What is the likely cause of this abdominal swelling?
(b) What would be the characteristic features on abdominal examination?
(c) What ancillary test would help to confirm the diagnosis?
(d) What should be done at operation?

124 (a) Describe the obstetrical landmarks noted in these views of a fetal skull.
(b) What are the presenting diameters in a vertex presentation?
(c) How do the presenting diameters of a face presentation differ?
(d) Comment on moulding of the head in labour.

124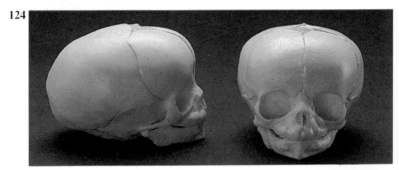

125 (a) What is the presentation of this fetus?
(b) What is the presenting diameter of this particular lie?
(c) What features would be recognised on vaginal examination?
(d) What is the preferred method of delivery?

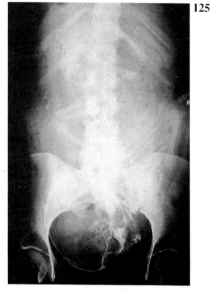

125

126 (a) What CTG abnormality is demonstrated?
(b) Describe the features of this abnormality.
(c) What is the implication of such a trace?
(d) What is the physiological basis for this abnormality?

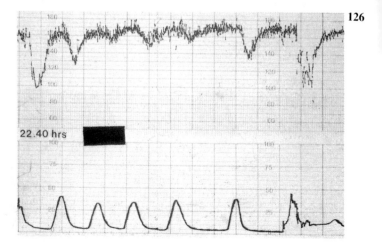

126

22.40 hrs

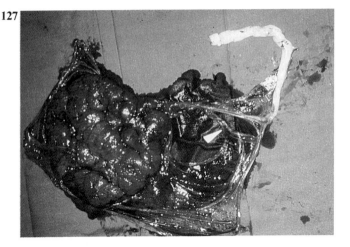

127,128 (a) What abnormality is demonstrated?
(b) What complication is likely?
(c) How may it present?
(d) With this abnormality are any blood tests of particular relevance?

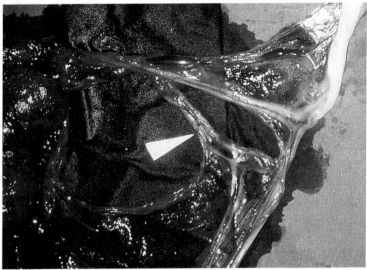

129 A 15-year-old girl attended with primary amenorrhoea and cyclical pelvic pain.
(a) What is the most likely diagnosis?
(b) What is the usual chromosomal pattern in this condition?
(c) What is the treatment of choice?
(d) Is there likely to be an associated abnormality of the genito-urinary tract?

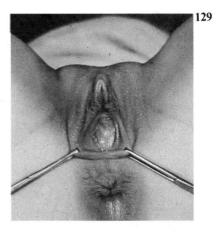

130 This child was born with a cloacal deformity.
(a) What is the basic reason for ambiguous genitalia?
(b) What drugs may cause virilisation of the female fetus when given to a pregnant woman?
(c) If the sex of the newborn infant is ambiguous what guideline should be used in assigning sex?
(d) If there is doubt about the fetal sex, when would a buccal smear be reliable?

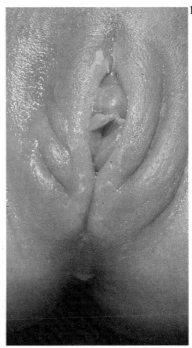

131

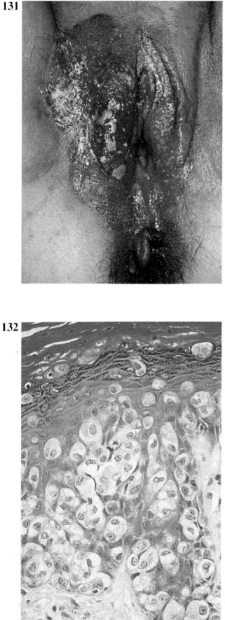

131,132 (a) From what condition is this patient suffering?
(b) What region of the vulva is affected by the lesion?
(c) What factors determine the outcome?
(d) What are characteristic features of the cells in **132**?

132

133 (a) What is the reason for the circular marking at the neck of this tumour?
(b) Has it been effective?
(c) What is the probable reason for the failure?
(d) Are these tumours likely to recur?

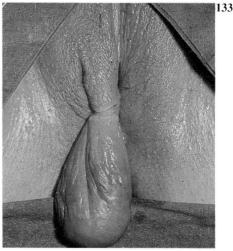

134 This is the appearance of a cervix following radical hysterectomy.
(a) Is the amount of vagina removed likely to be adequate?
(b) The patient, aged 25 years with a long history of infertility, became pregnant, and was then found to have abnormal cervical cytology. Further investigations revealed a microinvasive adeno-squamous carcinoma. At 16 weeks gestation, would it be justifiable to allow the pregnancy to continue?
(c) If the pregnancy continued, when should the patient be delivered?
(d) Would pelvic lymphadenectomy be indicated if a radical hysterectomy were performed?

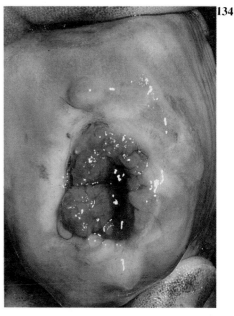

135

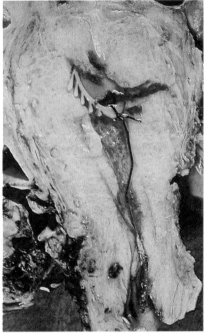

135 (a) What can be seen within this uterus?
(b) With what was this associated in particular?
(c) Why?
(d) What contraindications are there to fitting an IUCD?

136 (a) What is the condition shown in this biopsy taken from the cervix?
(b) Upon which part of the cervix does this condition develop?
(c) How does a patient with this condition usually present?
(d) Which factors place a patient at 'high risk' for the development of this condition?

136

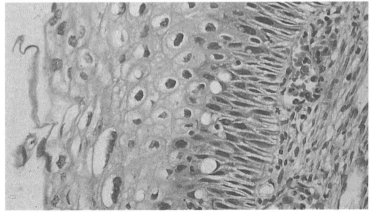

137 This 20-year-old patient presented with a 2-day history of a painful left vulval swelling.
(a) What is the diagnosis?
(b) What specific organism may be isolated?
(c) In what other ways may this infection present?
(d) How should it be treated?

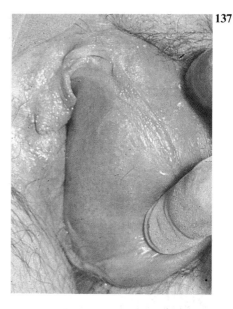

138 A carcinoma of the Fallopian tube is shown.
(a) How does it present?
(b) What is the patient's probable age?
(c) What is the treatment?
(d) What is the incidence of disease?

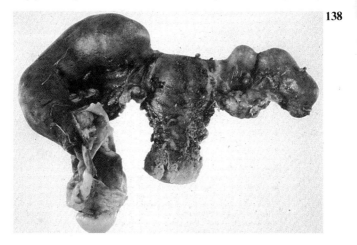

139

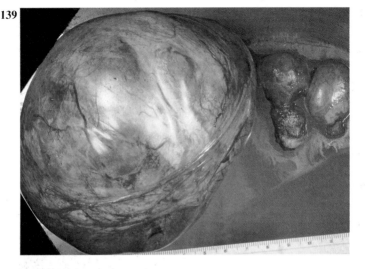

139 A 38-year-old asymptomatic patient was referred to the gynaecological clinic because of abdominal swelling. She had been told previously that she had fibroids and wondered if they had grown.
(a) Are the tumours removed ovarian or subserous fibroids?
(b) Was a hysterectomy necessary?
(c) In performing myomectomy operation, should the uterine cavity be opened and why?
(d) What are the chances of an ovarian cyst being malignant or a fibroid being malignant at this age?

140

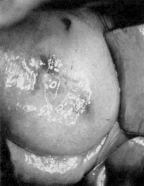

140 (a) What is the cervical lesion shown?
(b) Name the more common sites of this condition.
(c) In what ways may the condition present?
(d) What options are available in medical treatment of this condition?

141 The patient complained of vulval irritation but not of vaginal discharge. The appearance of the vagina on introducing a speculum is shown.

(a) What is the likely diagnosis?

(b) If the patient were 38 weeks pregnant what should be done?

(c) If the patient were menopausal, what other condition should be looked for or excluded?

(d) If some of the white plaques were dislodged, what would be seen?

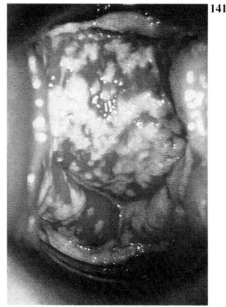

141

142 (a) What is a probable diagnosis?

(b) Suggest an alternative diagnosis.

(c) How should this condition be treated?

(d) Is it likely to be benign or malignant?

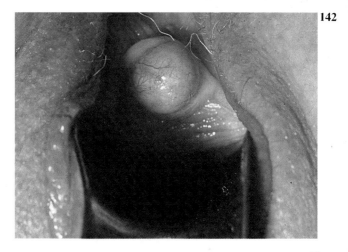

142

143

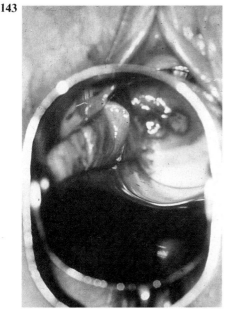

143 (a) What lesions are visible?
(b) What is the likely diagnosis?
(c) What is the responsible agent in the majority of cases?
(d) What is the usual time interval for occurrence of these lesions after exposure to this agent?

144

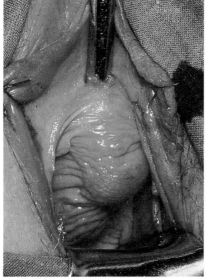

144 (a) What abnormality is present?
(b) Is it probably benign or malignant?
(c) How should it be treated?
(d) Is it likely to contain infective material?

145 Endometriosis in the vagina.
(a) Would this appearance be expected to change from time to time?
(b) What symptom would the patient probably complain of?
(c) How should she be treated medically?
(d) If treated surgically, could that be relied upon alone?

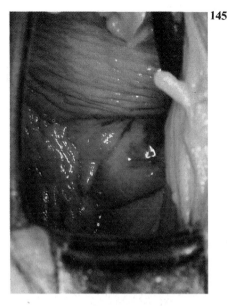

145

146 (a) Describe the histological changes shown in this cervical biopsy.
(b) How should the patient with this disease be investigated?
(c) What methods of treatment are available for this condition?
(d) If the patient were pregnant, how would this influence management?

146

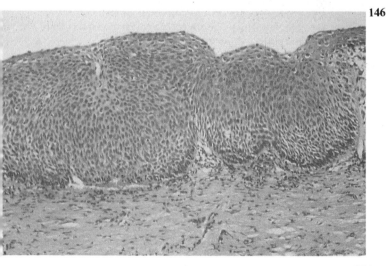

147

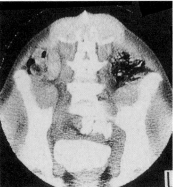

147 (a) Are these phaeochromocytoma easy to diagnose clinically in pregnancy?
(b) How would the suspected diagnosis be confirmed?
(c) Is there an increased risk with anaesthesia in such patients, if undiagnosed?
(d) What are the approximate risks of maternal death, if pregnant?

148,149 These photographs show a coronal CAT scan. **149** is an enlargement of an area from **148**.
(a) What is the opaque area in the pelvis?
(b) Is its outline normal?
(c) Is there any abnormality on the right pelvic wall?
(d) Is it possible to distinguish with certainty between lymph nodes enlarged due to infection and those due to malignancy?

148

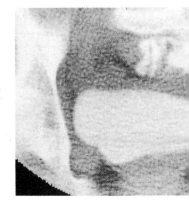

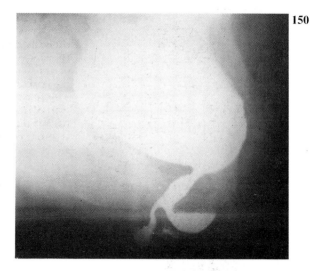

150 (a) What is this X-ray and what does it show?
(b) What is the possible aetiology?
(c) How may it present and what is the treatment?
(d) What other signs may it give in an X-ray?

151 (a) What is shown?
(b) What is the probable cause?
(c) What are the possible aetiological factors?
(d) What abdominal incision should be made to approach the pelvis in this patient?

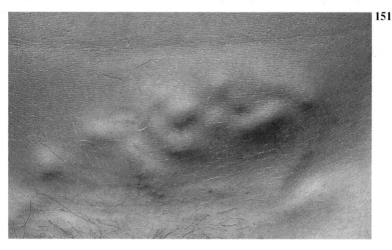

152

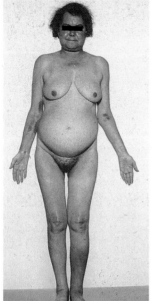

152 The patient complained of oligo-menorrhoea and infertility. In the course of investigations a blood cortisol level was reported as being greater than 15 μg/100 ml.
(a) What is a possible diagnosis?
(b) What test would verify the diagnosis?
(c) What would be the expected result of the test in this case?
(d) Is pregnancy possible with this condition?

153 (a) What is this?
(b) How would it be avoided?
(c) Which is preferable—unipolar or bipolar leads for surgical diathermy?
(d) Is high or low frequency electric current used?

153

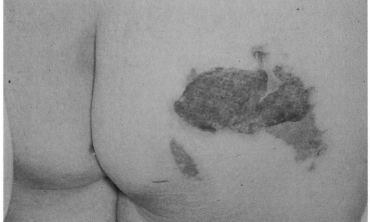

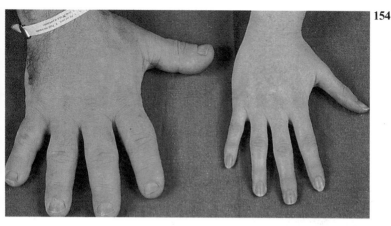

154 (a) From what condition is the patient on the left of the illustration suffering?
(b) How would such a patient most commonly present to the gynaecologist?
(c) How may the diagnosis be made in pregnancy?
(d) What is the usual pregnancy outcome?

155 The patient had a deep vein thrombosis in her pregnancy.
(a) What are the changes in the coagulation mechanisms which lead to an increased risk of thrombosis?
(b) What are other risk factors in pregnancy?
(c) What are the risks to the fetus from anticoagulant therapy?
(d) What are the maternal risks of long-term heparin therapy?

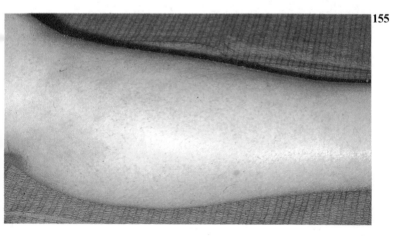

156

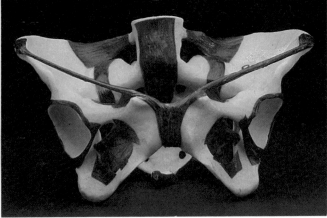

156,157 (a) Describe the features of this normal gynaecoid pelvis.
(b) In what percentage of women is such a pelvic type found?
(c) How does the android pelvis differ?
(d) In which clinical situations may pelvimetry be helpful in current obstetric practice?

157

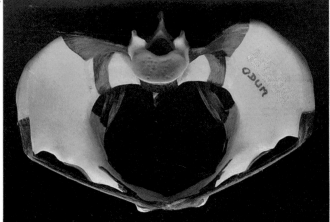

158 (a) Describe the features of this X-ray.
(b) What are the possible complications of this type of pregnancy?
(c) What are the characteristics of the placenta?
(d) What is the most common time of delivery?

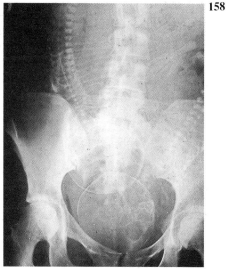

159 (a) Describe the placenta.
b) What is the term applied to the fetus in this illustration?
c) Is this a common condition?
d) What is the mechanism of the finding?

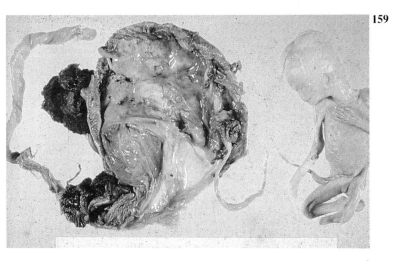

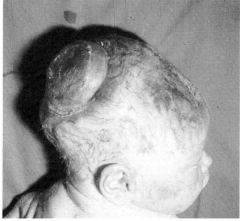

160 (a) By what technique has the baby been delivered?
(b) What are the potential hazards of this mode of delivery?
(c) What are the common indications for this procedure?
(d) What criteria must be met before using the technique?

161 (a) The diagnosis is straightforward but how should the patient be treated conservatively?
(b) Is it likely to be successful?
(c) Are these probably long-standing conditions?
(d) What operative procedures could be performed?

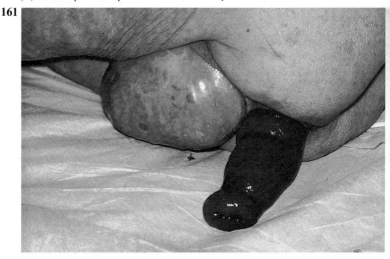

162 (a) From what medical condition does this patient suffer?
(b) What treatment should be recommended?
(c) Is there any justification for a vulval biospy?
(d) Would Ball's operation in which the nerve supply is divided be helpful to relieve symptoms?

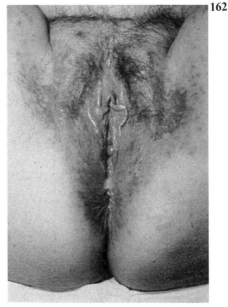

162

163 (a) What is the diagnosis?
(b) How would it be confirmed?
(c) What is the treatment?
(d) What is a more common site?

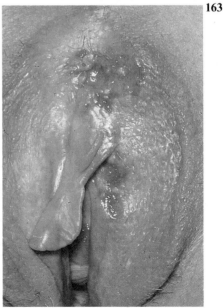

163

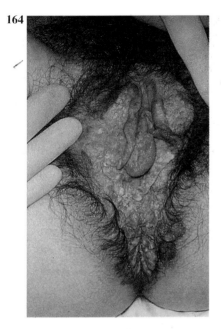

164 This is a Bowenoid lesion of the vulva.
(a) Describe the appearance of the lesion.
(b) What are the probable symptoms?
(c) If biopsies were taken, what features would be expected?
(d) In the modern classification of vulval dystrophies, would the term Bowen's disease be appropriate?

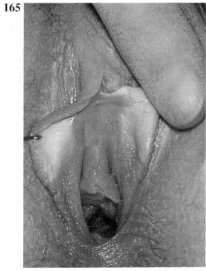

165 (a) If this were an incidental finding during routine gynaecological examination of a patient in her reproductive years what would be advisable?
(b) In a symptomless patient, is a biopsy justified?
(c) If classifying it as a dystrophy, how would it be described, hypertrophic or hypotrophic?
(d) Would it be associated with Candida infection?

166 (a) Was the patient from whom this uterus was removed premenopausal or postmenopausal?
(b) What was likely to be the predominant symptom?
(c) Would any particular operative risk be associated with removal of this uterus?
(d) What would the histology reveal?

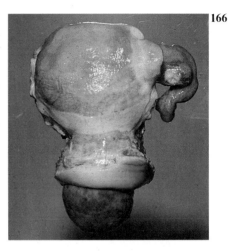

167 (a) Comment upon the specimen in the syringe obtained from this tubo-ovarian mass.
(b) Can the ovarian cyst be identified as a particular type?
(c) Is the lesion likely to be bilateral?
(d) What would be the patient's age group?

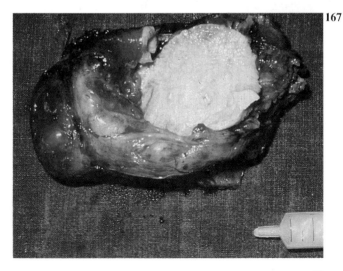

168

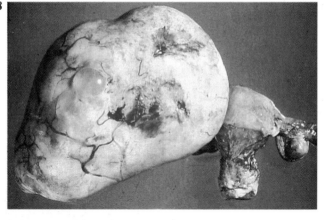

168 (a) In what age group was the woman from whom this specimen was taken?
(b) What would be the abdominal incision of choice to remove the specimen and why?
(c) What should be done on opening the peritoneal cavity?
(d) Is this the front or back view of the uterus?

169 (a) What features are shown?
(b) What is the differential diagnosis of this condition?
(c) What blood test would help to elucidate the cause?
(d) If constitutional, what drug might help?

169

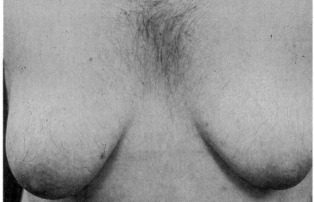

170 A superficial ulcer in the vagina which was painful and tender is shown.
(a) What is the likely diagnosis?
(b) How is the diagnosis established in the laboratory?
(c) For how long are the ulcers infectious?
(d) Can transmission occur with asymptomatic lesions?

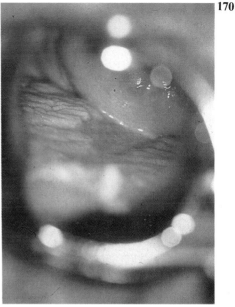

171 (a) What is shown on this X-ray?
(b) What other investigations may be useful?
(c) What treatment should be given?
(d) If contraceptive advice is requested, what should be suggested?

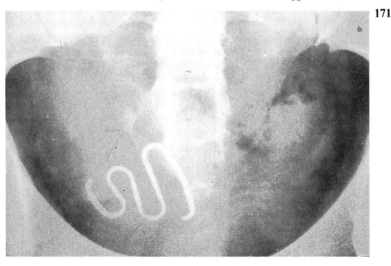

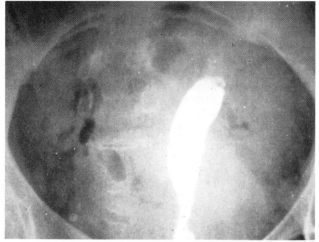

172 (a) What is the abnormality shown?
(b) Is any other investigation justified and if so, which?
(c) What other abnormality might be found?
(d) What is the probable state of the Fallopian tubes and ovaries?

173 (a) What is this instrument?
(b) What is the purpose of the camera?
(c) What is the purpose of the extended single eyepiece?
(d) What is the advantage of this apparatus?

173

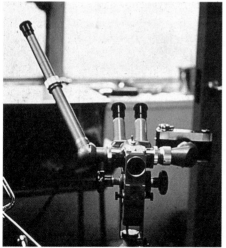

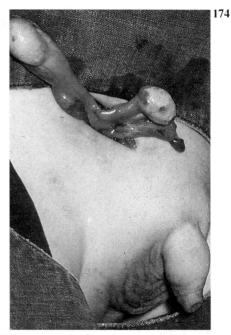

174,175 (a) Is it possible to tell from **174** whether this patient is a true hermaphrodite?
(b) Does **175** indicate some Mullerian duct tissue?
(c) Would the gonads be testes, ovaries, ovotestes or a mixture?
(d) Would a Y chromosome be expected to be present?

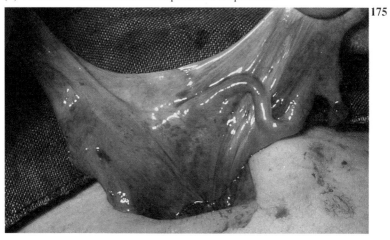

176

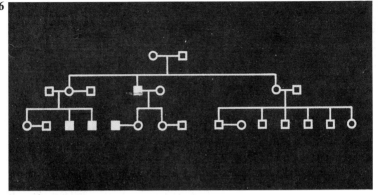

176 Which of the following conditions would be expected to conform to the pattern of inheritance shown?
(a) Haemophilia A (Classical).
(b) Phenylketonuria.
(c) Myotonic dystrophy.
(d) Tay-Sachs disease.

177 (a) What is the cardiotographic abnormality shown?
(b) What are maternal causes of this change?
(c) What are fetal causes of this change?
(d) What are the drug causes of this change?

177

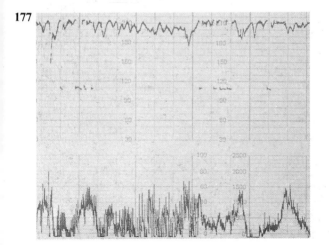

178 This tissue was passed when a patient had a spontaneous abortion.

(a) What is the diagnosis?

(b) What is the usual subsequent clinical course?

(c) Which clinical factors are associated with a high risk of malignant sequelae?

(d) The beta HCG level falls to normal within a few weeks but when should it be regarded as abnormal?

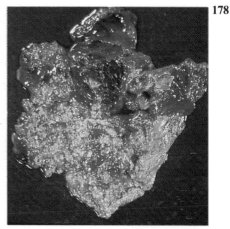

179 (a) What abnormalities are seen in these amniotic bands?

(b) What is the presumed cause of amniotic bands?

(c) What fetal anomalies are associated with amniotic bands?

(d) Are amniotic bands immediately evident?

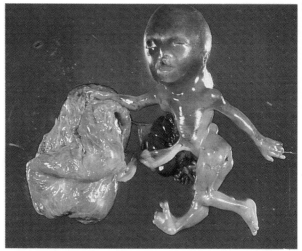

180

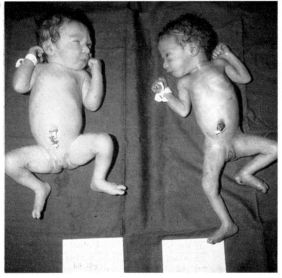

180 These babies are uniovular twins.
(a) What is the reason for the discrepancy in their appearance?
(b) What proportion of twins are binovular?
(c) What is the frequency of two chorions with monozygotic twinning?
(d) What factors influence the incidence of dizygotic twins?

181

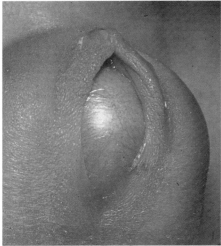

181 (a) This is not what it appears to be! What is the more common diagnosis?
(b) What is shown?
(c) Are the two conditions managed in a similar manner?
(d) Does the less common condition occur at an earlier or later age than the more common condition?

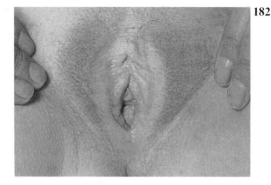

182 This lesion was noted in a 7-year-old girl and was reviewed regularly. However, vulval irritation became intense and she was admitted for a vulval biopsy.
(a) What would be the diagnosis after vulval biopsy?
(b) Is it likely to get better spontaneously?
(c) To relieve the child's symptoms, what treatment should be given?
(d) What percentage of postmenopausal patients with this condition may develop malignant change?

183 (a) What is this condition?
(b) What other areas are likely to be affected?
(c) Is it infectious?
(d) What is the treatment?

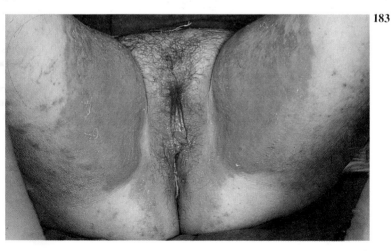

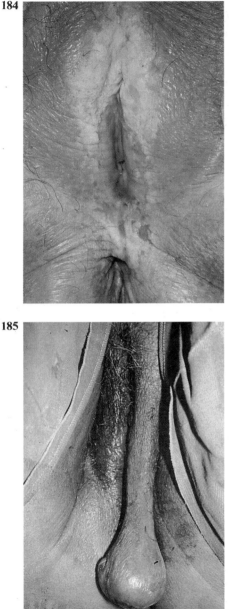

184 A vulval dystrophy is shown.

(a) How could the patient's symptoms be relieved?

(b) How often should the patient be seen?

(c) If the lesion remained clinically unchanged, would vulval biopsies be indicated from time to time and, if so, how often?

(d) How would this dystrophy be classified?

185 (a) What is this?

(b) How would it present?

(c) What complications may occur?

(d) What treatment should be performed?

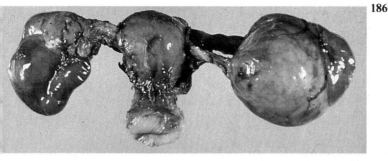

186 This 40-year-old patient had several attacks of pelvic inflammatory disease and increasingly heavy and frequent periods. The only way to relieve her symptoms was a total hysterectomy conserving one or both of the ovaries, if possible. She had previously had a làparotomy through a Pfannenstiel incision.
(a) Was it possible to conserve the ovaries?
(b) On histological examination if one of the ovaries were found to contain a cystadenocarcinoma what should be advised?
(c) Under these circumstances should hormone replacement therapy be given?
(d) In the presence of bilateral swellings, possibly tubo-ovarian pre-operatively, what abdominal incision should be used?

187 (a) What abnormal feature is shown?
(b) What is the aetiology?
(c) What investigations should be recommended?
(d) In the absence of cervical intraepithelial neoplasia (CIN) what should be recommended?

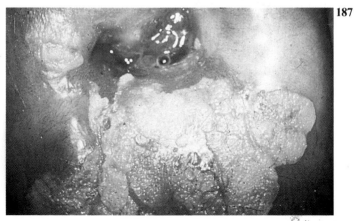

188

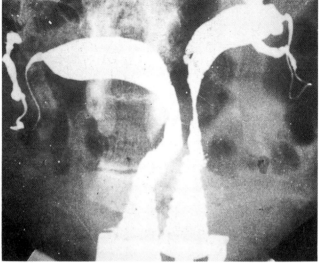

188,189 (a) Compare and contrast these two hysterosalpingograms by defining the characteristic features.
(b) What is the embryological basis of these findings?
(c) At what gestation does this occur?
(d) Which of the women with these X-ray findings is more likely to have obstetric complications?

189

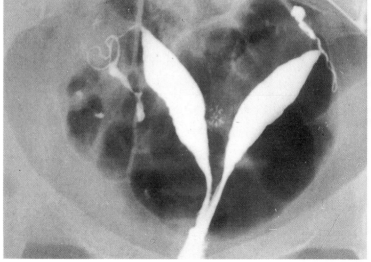

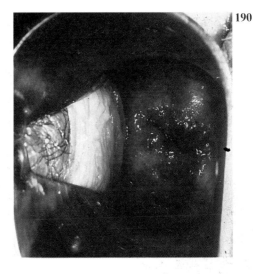

190 This photograph was taken during the examination of a 'well woman' who had never had a cervical cytology smear.

a) Does the cervix appear healthy and why?

b) If the woman is symptomless, and a cervical smear taken during the examination is subsequently reported as normal, what should be done?

c) When should a repeat smear be taken?

191 The patient has secondary syphilis.

a) When does the rash generally appear?

b) Is it associated with lymphadenopathy?

c) Can the lesions be limited to the genitalia only?

d) If undiagnosed in pregnancy what would be the likely outcome for the fetus?

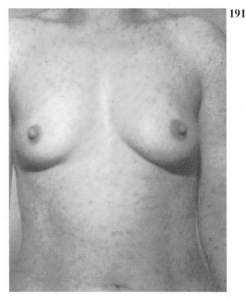

192

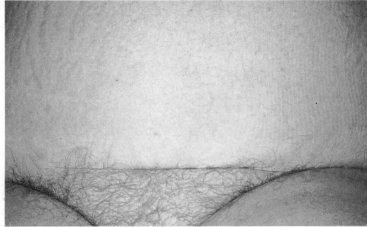

192 (a) What are the characteristics of this condition (*Peau d'orange*) and by what mechanism does it occur?
(b) Why did it occur in this patient?
(c) What other signs or symptoms may she have?
(d) Had she any previous operations?

193 (a) What clinical sign does the patient demonstrate?
(b) Which drug is commonly associated with this condition?
(c) What are the risks to the fetus for a patient receiving this drug?
(d) What other state may produce similar features?

193

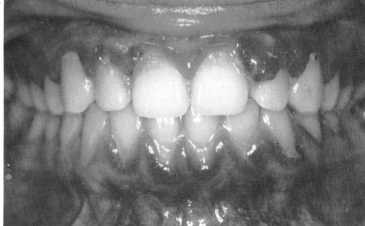

194 (a) What are these vulval lesions?
(b) Are they infective?
(c) What other signs and symptoms may be present?
(d) What blood tests will confirm the diagnosis?

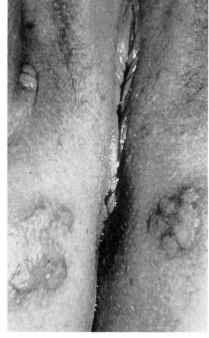

195 (a) What is the name given to this method of assessing fetal well-being?
(b) What instruction should be given to the mother regarding the recording of activity?
(c) When should she report to her doctor or midwife?
(d) What additional assessment should then be undertaken?

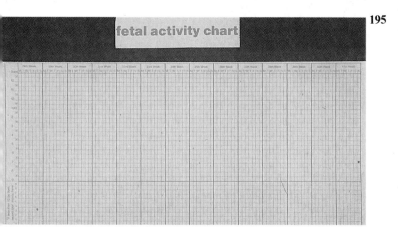

196

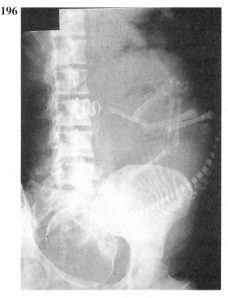

196 (a) What does this X-ray reveal?

(b) What associated complications may occur in early pregnancy?

(c) What recommendations should be made for the conduct of delivery?

(d) What form of contraception should be recommended?

197 (a) What CTG abnormality is demonstrated?

(b) Of what significance is such a pattern?

(c) In association with what underlying fetal condition is this described?

(d) What is the management i) antenatally; ii) in labour?

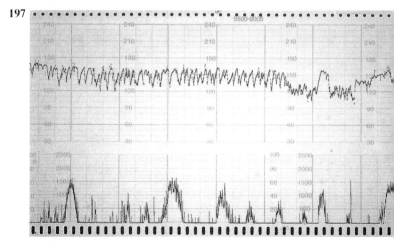

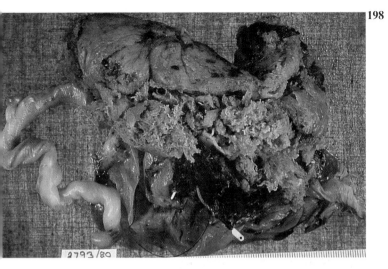

198

198 (a) What abnormality can be seen?
(b) What is the incidence of pregnancy with an IUCD *in situ*?
(c) What are the complications of pregnancy with an IUCD *in situ*?
(d) How is an IUCD *in situ* best managed in early pregnancy?

199 (a) What abnormality does this baby have?
(b) What is the common association?
(c) How may this abnormality be predicted antenatally?
(d) What is the background incidence in the United Kingdom?

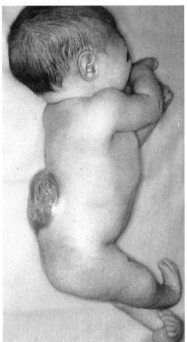

199

200

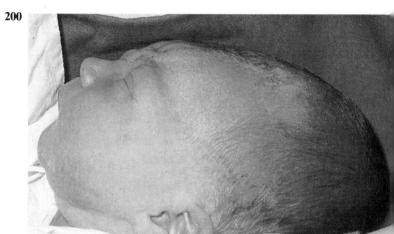

200 (a) What is the usual cause of a cepalohaematoma?
(b) What is a second possible cause?
(c) What is the usual site?
(d) What is the normal progress?

201

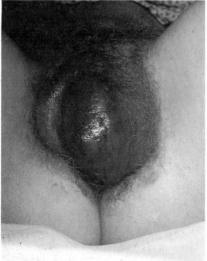

201 (a) What is the diagnosis?
(b) Give an account of a common type of acciden which is associated with thi finding.
(c) Are there usually any long term sequelae?
(d) In this the type of injury which occurs in rape?

202 This is the typical appearance of severe vulval dystrophy.
(a) What would be the two main complaints of this patient?
(b) What is her age group?
(c) Is she likely to be cured?
(d) What is the term which was often applied to this condition?

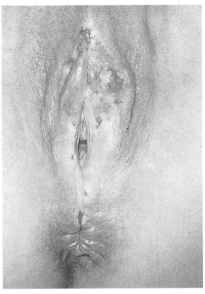

203 (a) What is the problem in this 3-year-old child?
(b) How could it be prevented from happening again?
(c) Can this condition be treated as an outpatient?
(d) To what is it sometimes secondary?

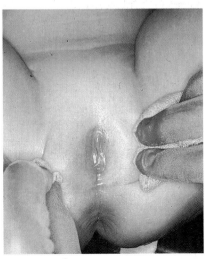

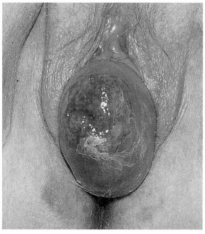

204 This patient complained of a 'lump down below'.
(a) What is the diagnosis?
(b) If she had suffered a recent myocardial infarct, how should she be treated?
(c) If the patient were fit for operation, which procedure should be followed?
(d) What is the chance of this patient having stress incontinence?

205 A serous cystadenoma of the ovary, removed from a 38-year-old patient.
(a) In which age group does this commonly occur?
(b) Although unilateral in this case, what proportion are bilateral?
(c) What percentage are likely to become malignant?
(d) Is any feature associated with a greater possibility of their being bilateral or becoming malignant?

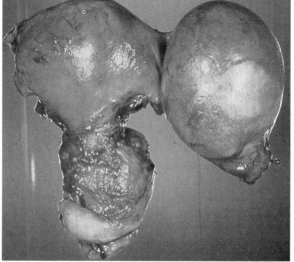

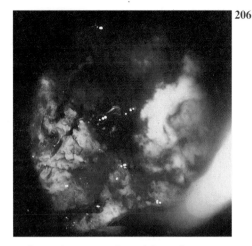

206 After two abnormal smears, the patient was referred for colposcopy. Saline has been applied to the cervix and the magnification is × 100.
a) What is the purpose of using saline?
b) Is any additional help required if the saline technique is used?
c) Although obscured by blood in many areas, is there an obvious abnormality?
d) What other solutions may be applied to the cervix and how are the abnormal areas identified?

207 (a) What abnormality can be seen?
b) How may this present?
c) If diagnosed during labour what action should be taken?
d) What other developmental abnormalities may be associated?

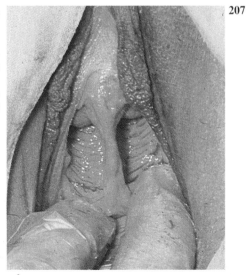

208

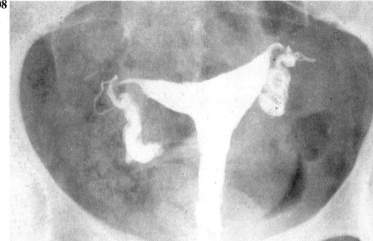

208 (a) What investigation has been carried out?
(b) What is the result?
(c) What further investigations should be offered?
(d) What treatment might be appropriate?

209 (a) What is the abnormality shown?
(b) Could it be prevented?
(c) Is dental caries aggravated by pregnancy?
(d) Is dental repair and extraction safe during pregnancy?

209

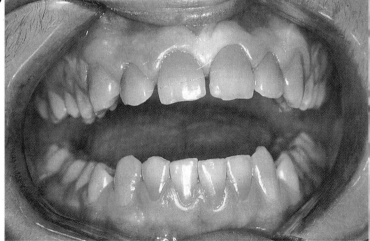

210 (a) What is the presentation of this fetus?
(b) What technique may be considered with a view to correcting this malpresentation?
(c) What are the contraindications to this procedure?
(d) What steps should be taken following the procedure?

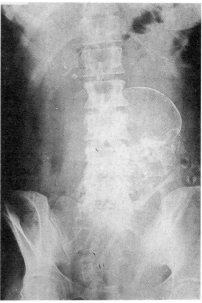

211 (a) What type of placenta is shown?
(b) What is the incidence of the associated pregnancy?
(c) What is the ratio of 'zygosity' in these pregnancies?
(d) What are possible predisposing factors?

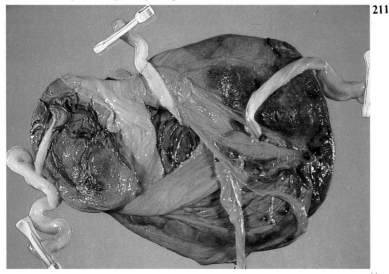

212

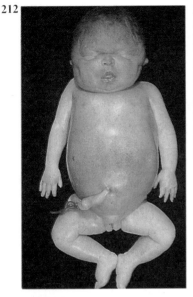

212 (a) The appearance of this infant results from a blood group incompatibility between mother and fetus. Why have such infants become rare in present times?
(b) Why are some infants with this appearance still seen?
(c) Does the disease process follow the same pattern in subsequent pregnancies?
(d) Name some alternative causes for infants with this appearance.

213 (a) Describe the features shown by this neonate.
(b) What is the name given to this condition and what is the underlying abnormality?
(c) How may this present antenatally?
(d) What is the prognosis?

213

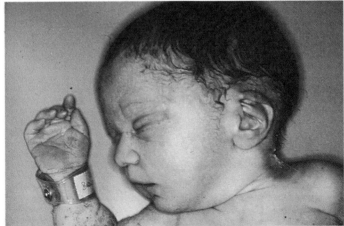

214 (a) What is the probable cause of these ulcers?
(b) Which is the most common site to be involved?
(c) From which maternal site does the neonate most commonly acquire infection during delivery?
(d) What treatment could be suggested for the vulval lesions?

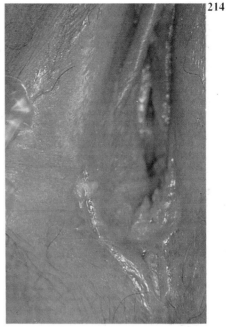

214

215 (a) What is the diagnosis in this elderly patient?
(b) How should it be treated?
(c) What histological type of tumour would be expected?
(d) Since the prolapse had been present for a long time, what new symptom would have brought the patient back to the doctor?

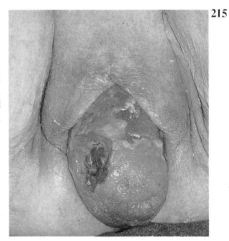

215

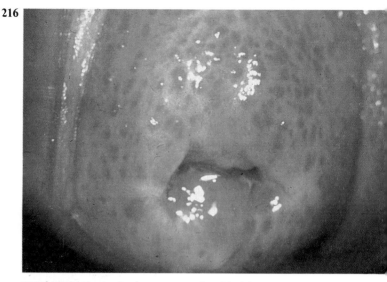

216 (a) What name is given to a cervix with this appearance?
(b) What infective organism is usually responsible?
(c) What are the morphological features of the responsible organism?
(d) What is the treatment of choice?

217 (a) What is the likely diagnosis?
(b) What are the clinical features of the condition?
(c) What biochemical investigations would be helpful?
(d) What are the probable findings on examination of the breasts?

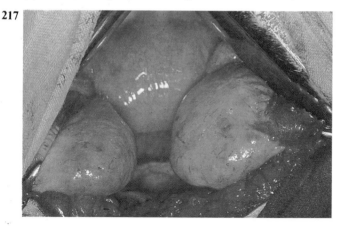

218 This 20-year-old patient complained of primary amenorrhoea and had a 15-year-old sister who had not yet menstruated.
a) What is the likely diagnosis and how could it be confirmed?
b) What would probably be found on bimanual examination?
c) What treatment would be suggested?
d) What is the aetiology of the condition?

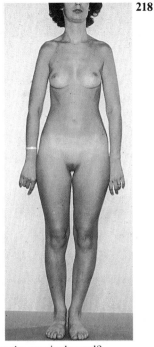

218

219 This patient was referred for colposcopy following two abnormal smears. Schiller's test indicates the glycogen-free areas.
a) Is it possible to exclude a lesion extending up the cervical canal?
b) Where should the biopsies be taken, using the cervix as the face of a clock?
c) Could biopsies be taken without using a colposcope?
d) Is there any advantage to biopsy under colposcopic control?

219

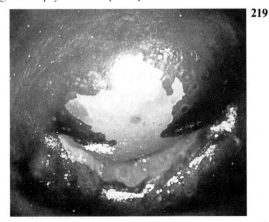

ANSWERS

(a) A right mediolateral episiotomy.
(b) Prevention of lacerations especially third degree tear; prevention of damage to the neonate—it shortens second stage, and is helpful in the prevention of subsequent pelvic floor relaxation.
(c) Extension of the incision; increased blood loss; pain; infection and dyspareunia.
(d) Midline or J-shaped.

2 (a) Shoulder dystocia.
(b) Diabetic mothers.
(c) Erb's palsy caused by brachial plexus injury.
(d) Cephalic (left-occipito-anterior).

3 (a) Amniocentesis—to collect amniotic fluid for estimation of the bilirubin level.
(b) Ultrasound for assessment of growth; check fetus for oedema or ascites.
(c) Diagnosis of fetal chromosome, biochemical, enzyme and neural tube abnormalities. Lecithin/sphingomyelin ratio for fetal lung maturity.
(d) Abortion or premature labour; ruptured membranes feto-maternal transfusion, amniotic bands or minor limb deformity.

4 (a) Complete hydatidiform mole.
(b) With hyperemesis, pre-eclampsia, passage of vesicles, and the uterus not consistent with dates. Absence of fetal movements, fetal parts and fetal heart on examination. Thyrotoxicosis occasionally may be present.
(c) 46 XX—both of paternal origin.
(d) All patients should be registered and followed up with serial human chorionic gonadotrophin estimations for at least 1 and preferably 2 years. Pregnancy should be avoided for the same period.

5 (a) Serum prolactin—where elevation would indicate a possible pituitary tumour.
(b) An X-ray of the pituitary fossa and possibly tomography or CAT scan of the fossa.
(c) Bromocriptine.
(d) Removal or ablation of the pituitary tumour.

6 (a) Donovanosis (granuloma inguinale).
(b) Carcinoma of the vulva.
(c) Smear and/or biopsy for Donovan bodies and a biopsy of the lesion for carcinoma of the vulva.
(d) Yes. It may develop while ulceration is still active or after the ulcers have healed.

7,8 (a) Donovan bodies.
(b) Calymmatobacterium granulomatis (formerly Donovania granulomatis).
(c) Skin and mucous membranes.
(d) Mouth, nose or pharynx.

9 (a) Yes, if lymphatic obstruction is the cause and it remains uncorrected, otherwise surgical removal should be effective.
(b) Filariasis, tuberculous adenitis and lymphogranuloma venereum.
(c) Malignant growths, secondary syphilis and Donovanosis (granuloma inguinale)—the diagnosis in this patient.
(d) Most ulcers are painful or itchy and in Donovanosis quite tender to touch.

10 (a) It appears pigmented like a melanoma, but could be old blood within a haemangioma. It was a melanoma.
(b) Biopsy or biopsy excision.
(c) It is directly related to the depth of invasion.
(d) Those where the invasion of the melanoma only involves the intra papillary ridge.

11 (a) Large fibroid uterus with both adnexae attached.
(b) Hyaline, cystic, calcification, necrosis, red degeneration and sarcomatous change (rare).
(c) Heavy periods, pain, a mass or swelling noted and urinary symptoms.
(d) At least 45 years because the ovaries have been removed.

12 (a) Laparoscopes × 2; Verres' needles × 2; aspiration needles; Bard Parker scalpel handle and blade; trochars and cannulae × 2; Michel clip applicator; Currie's cannula and methylene blue dye in syringe; Volsellum forceps.
(b) Pencil pointed trochar.
(c) Carbon dioxide or nitrous oxide.
(d) Palmer forceps (or Drapier forceps) if using diathermy, Hulka-Clemens clips, Filshie clips or Falope rings, with their applicators, trochars and cannulae.

13 (a) Haematosalpinx due to ectopic pregnancy.
(b) Amenorrhoea, symptoms of early pregnancy, abdominal pain, vaginal bleeding.
(c) Unilateral adnexal tenderness, cervical excitation, bulky uterus and occasionally a mass may be felt.
(d) Urinary pregnancy test, serum beta human chorionic gonadotrophin ultrasound scan and laparoscopy, unless the diagnosis is obvious.

14 (a) Uterus, vagina, rectum, anus, Fallopian tube.
(b) Posterior exenteration.
(c) As a curative procedure for carcinoma of the posterior vaginal wall without metastases, or for central recurrent disease following radiotherapy.
(d) Upper vagina—cervical lymphatic distribution.
Lower third of vagina—vulval lymphatic distribution.

15 (a) Graafian follicle.
(b) FSH/LH from the anterior pituitary; FSH/LH releasing hormones from the hypothalamus and oestrogen from the follicles.
(c) Rupture to release an ovum; the follicle then forms a corpus luteum. The majority of follicles cease development before this and become atretic.
(d) Primary oocyte 48, secondary 24.

16 (a) Fibroid polyp.
(b) Sarcoma, endometrial carcinoma, products of conception and uterine inversion.
(c) Examination under anaesthesia, ligation and division of the fibroid pedicle, then pathological confirmation of the diagnosis.
(d) If the lesion is sarcomatous, then radical surgery may not necessarily improve the prognosis. Nevertheless, standard treatment would involve total abdominal hysterectomy and bilateral salpingo-oophorectomy (although the need for oophorectomy is controversial). Chemotherapy has limited benefit if any.

17 (a) A urethral caruncle.
(b) Urethral prolapse (ie circumferential prolapse) or urethral carcinoma.
(c) Angiomatous, polypoid and granulomatous type of urethral caruncle.
(d) Radiotherapy with an interstitial source.

18,19 (a) Vaginal adenosis.
(b) Whether the patient's mother took drugs during pregnancy to prevent spontaneous abortion, notably diethylstiboestrol (DES).
(c) Vaginal adenosis is present in about 85 per cent of women exposed to DES in utero.
(d) Probably a maximum incidence of 1 in 1000 exposed females.

20 (a) Appearance is suggestive of trichomonas vaginalis but as patient has salpingitis, a gonococcal infection is also possible.
(b) High vaginal swabs, cervical, urethral, rectal and pharyngeal swabs should be obtained and cultured.
(c) Tests for the exclusion of syphilis and also a white cell count and ESR.
(d) Penicillin and metronidazole.

21 (a) Bilateral wedge resection of ovaries.
(b) Reduction of the amount of ovarian tissue which should reduce the androgen/oestrogen imbalance.
(c) Possibility of developing tubal adhesions which may be a subsequent factor in infertility.
(d) Prednisolone, plus clomiphene or tamoxifen, gonadotrophin therapy.

22 (a) Osteoporosis.
(b) An essential feature of osteoporosis is loss of bone mass. This results from bone reabsorption exceeding bone formation.
(c) Physical activity appears to slow down the process of bone loss and demineralisation.
(d) It is reputed to be a major factor predisposing to osteoporosis.

23 (a) An intrauterine conraceptive device (IUCD).
(b) Copper 7.
(c) Low down on the side of the uterus just above the left ovary there appears to be a perforation site through which the IUCD may have travelled.
(d) It is important for future attendants to be aware of a previous uterine perforation, although it is unlikely to cause complications in subsequent pregnancies.

24 (a) Yes, to the right ovary which is enlarged.
(b) In the postmenopausal period.
(c) Adenocarcinoma.
(d) The poor prognosis reflects the difficulty in making a diagnosis and the fact that it is made at a late stage.

25 (a) Fibroids (leiomyomata).
(b) In the broad ligament.
(c) Yes, the left ureter.
(d) An abdominal swelling or mass.

26 (a) Chorea gravidarum.
(b) Facial grimacing and choreic posture of hands.
(c) Most authorities now agree it is identical with Sydenham's (rheumatic) chorea, having the same uncertain cause.
(d) Yes, it has a tendency to recur although the condition itself is relatively uncommon.

27 (a) Herpes gestationis.
(b) Pruritus.
(c) Prednisolone usually brings prompt relief and inhibits the formation of the new lesions. Pyridoxine has also been used and appears to be effective in some cases.
(d) Yes, this has been reported and also that the lesions clear spontaneously during the neonatal period.

28,29 (a) Haematocolpos, and possibly an associated haematometra to account for the abdominal swelling.
(b) Following puberty, retained menstrual loss caused cyclical abdominal pain and urinary symptoms in association with amenorrhoea. An abdominal swelling may eventually appear.
(c) Transverse vaginal membranes—usually distinct from the hymen. Occasionally, the vagina may be imperforate for some distance.
(d) Incision of the imperforate membrane and drainage of the haematocolpos, sometimes under antibiotic cover.

30 (a) From the top: diaphragm, Multiload intrauterine contraceptive device (IUCD), and Gravigard (Copper 7) IUCD.
(b) 10–15 per 100 woman-years, to which poor patient compliance may contribute.
(c) Approximately 3 per 100 woman-years.
(d) Expulsion, perforation, heavier and more painful menses and increase in the relative risk factor for pelvic infection and ectopic pregnancy.

31 (a) Hydrocephalic fetus presenting by the frank breech.
(b) An open spina bifida may be recognised.
(c) Obstruction at delivery of the head.
(d) Decompression of the fetal head by drainage of cerebrospinal fluid. If the head had been presenting, the CSF could have been drained off abdominally after using local infiltration of the skin or vaginally if the membranes had ruptured.

32 (a) Prolonged pregnancy.
(b) Dry flaking skin and lack of vernix.
(c) Uteroplacental insufficiency resulting in fetal hypoxia and ultimately fetal death in utero, meconium aspiration and reduction in the ability of the fetal skull to mould.
(d) The placenta may show calcification and/or infarcts but in the majority of cases appears macroscopically normal.

33 (a) Type 1 dips or early decelerations.
(b) Continued cardiotocographic recording. In the presence of meconium stained liquor or other features of fetal compromise, fetal blood sampling would be appropriate.
(c) No.
(d) No.

34 (a) A placenta with velamentous insertion of the cord.
(b) Vasa praevia.
(c) Vessels may be palpated within the membranes, ahead of the presenting part. Compression of these vessels may cause sudden alteration in the fetal heart rate pattern. If the vessels rupture there will be bleeding of fetal origin with acute fetal distress.
(d) If there is intrapartum bleeding, the presence of fetal blood can be confirmed by the alkali denaturation test (Singer's test or Apt's test). This depends upon the fact that fetal haemoglobin is more resistant to denaturation by alkali than adult haemoglobin.

35 (a) Bilateral hydronephrosis.
(b) Hydroureter.
(c) Yes.
(d) No, it would depend upon the clinical presentation of the patient.

36 (a) Herpes genitalis.
(b) Pain or retention of urine.
(c) Swabs from the lesions transported to the laboratory in viral culture medium. Check for other forms of sexually transmitted diseases and secondary infection.
(d) Commonly sexually transmitted; the incubation period is 3–7 days. Recurrent attacks are often at menses. Severity and frequency of attacks may be reduced by antiviral agents. — *Acyclovir*

37 (a) This is a skin deposit of chronic myeloid leukaemia. Blood count and film is likely to suggest the diagnosis. White blood counts are usually above $30,000/mm^3$ (commonly $100,000–125,000/mm^3$), and a whole range of immature granulocytes may be seen in the film. The patient may be anaemic.
(b) Biopsy for histology of the lesion and bone marrow studies.
(c) Treatment of the primary disorder, usually be chemotherapy, although radiotherapy, splenectomy and marrow transplant may have a part to play.
(d) The Philadelphia chromosome which involves translocation of genetic material from the long arm of one chromosome, 22 usually to chromosome 9. This is found in leukaemia precursor cells.

38 (a) Yes, one side is commonly more affected than the other.
(b) Ulceration.
(c) Yes, but often there is only unilateral lymph node involvement.
(d) Tuberculosis.

39,40 (a) A polyp arising from the cervix.
(b) Excision biopsy and curettage to exclude any uterine polyp.
(c) Diathermy or ligation if base of pedicle is accessible.
(d) Trauma.

41 (a) Human tubercle (mycobacterium tuberculosis) bacillus is the likely cause. Confirm by culture and/or guinea pig inoculation.
(b) Infertility, secondary amenorrhoea, ectopic pregnancy, intermenstrual discharge, pain, malaise, but rarely weight loss.
(c) Via the blood stream from lungs, lymph nodes, renal tract and bones. Direct or lymphatic spread from adjacent pelvic organs. Rarely ascending from a primary site on vulva, vagina or cervix.
(d) Antituberculous drugs. Surgery rarely may be considered nowadays and only if there is inadequate response to chemotherapy.

42 (a) Dyspnoea and pain in the chest.
(b) A pulmonary embolus removed at the time of a Trendelenburg operation.
(c) Barrier methods would be preferable.
(d) Prophylactic anticoagulant therapy but deep vein thrombosis and/or pulmonary embolism may still recur, as happened in this patient.

43 (a) Principally in older women with the peak incidence around 70 years of age.
(b) Vaginal bleeding, abdominal pain and vaginal discharge.
(c) Yes.
(d) From indifferent Mullerian mesenchymal cells which differentiate into both epithelial and stromal elements.

44 (a) In 1968 there was a single peak of age-incidence at about 50 years but a change had occurred by 1979 to produce almost two peaks, one at 30–35 and one at 55–60 years.
(b) The incidence of carcinoma of the cervix in younger women has increased.

(c) It possibly reflects changing sexual practices and the use of non-barrier methods of contraception..

(d) Yes, the fall in the number of cases of carcinoma of the cervix in older women almost certainly reflects this.

45 (a) Dullness to percussion is most marked in the flanks with ascites whereas it may be central with a cyst. Hamilton Bailey recommended pressing a ruler across the swelling, because a giant cyst will transmit aortic pulsation whereas ascites will not.

(b) Ultrasound will show omentum and bowel within ascites, whereas a cyst will contain no bowel.

(c) Benign.

(d) Surgery should be performed to include a total abdominal hysterectomy, bilateral salpingo-oophorectomy, omentectomy and assessment of the entire peritoneal cavity for signs of spread. Biopsies of any suspicious lesions and peritoneal washings should be taken. Chemotherapy may be indicated.

46 (a) Cervical mucus sampling.

(b) Ferning on slide, or production of spinnbarkeit.

(c) Presence of secretory IgA antibodies to sperm, abnormally low pH.

(d) Post-coital test, sperm–mucous penetration test, eg Kremer test involving cross-over testing with donor sperm and mucus.

47 (a) Nabothian cyst (follicle) on the cervix.

(b) The result of mucus distension of the endocervical glands.

(c) In the majority of cases, no.

(d) They can be evacuated with diathermy, cautery or cryosurgery.

48 (a) Malignant.

(b) Secondary.

(c) Adenocarcinoma; more likely than squamous. Sarcoma is also a possibility.

(d) Poor if secondary, especially if a sarcoma (which it is). There is a better albeit poor, outlook if this is a metastasis from an endometrial carcinoma.

49,50 (a) There is a large fistula involving bladder neck and proximal urethra. Note the small quantity of urine in the vagina.

(b) Obstructed labour. Fistulae close to the cervix may follow trauma at Caesarean section.

(c) Schistosomiasis and tuberculosis.

(d) Surgical repair by a vaginal approach. Longitudinal repair gives a better chance of urethral function. If there is much tissue loss, then transverse closure may be necessary to avoid tension in the tissues which would lead to failure of the repair. A Martius graft (a pedicle graft of subcutaneous fat from the labium majus) may be used to reinforce the repair, ensure mobility of the bladder neck and fill potential dead space.

51 (a) A double uterus, which is bicornis unicollis.

(b) Intravenous pyelogram for associated congenital abnormalities of the urinary tract.

(c) There is often a band from the bladder to the rectum. This should be divided prior to the hysterectomy. Care should also be taken with the ureters.

(d) Strassman's operation (uteroplasty).

52 (a) Asia, Africa and Latin America.

(b) About 50 per cent.

(c) Less than 35 years.

(d) About 90 per cent.

53 (a) Vulval intraepithelial neoplasia, grade III, with microinvasion shown in the centre.
(b) It is reported with increasing frequency in younger women.
(c) Preclinical or clinical neoplasia in about 12 per cent of patients in other sites of the anogenital epithelium. The majority of these lesions will be found on the cervix.
(d) The depth of invasion, the degree of differentiation and the presence of vascular space involvement influence the chance of regional node metastasis and, hence, prognosis.

54 (a) A large solid mass in the pelvis and lower abdomen as the iliac crest can be visualised and there is a lumbar vertebra posteriorly.
(b) Dermoid cyst (teratoma).
(c) Straight X-ray of the abdomen.
(d) Up to 5 per cent.

55 (a) Intra-abdominal pressure (either with a rectal, gastric or intra-peritoneal pressure transducer); intravesical pressure; detrusor pressure (produced by electronic subtraction of abdominal pressure from vesical pressure).
(b) No, normal bladder capacity is usually over 400–500 ml.
(c) No, it is usually greater than 150 ml. Such a low level may be due to urethral irritation by the catheter.
(d) Yes.

56 (a) Acute breast engorgement.
(b) The third to seventh day postpartum.
(c) Mastitis and breast abscess.
(d) Bromocriptine but this will suppress lactation. Oestrogens may be beneficial but are associated with a risk of thromboembolism.

57 (a) An enlarged left supraclavicular nodal mass.
(b) More likely to be malignant (although it could be either).
(c) No, as the enlarged nodes are too superficial to cause interference with the cervical sympathetic nerve fibres.
(d) Carcinoma of the cervix, endometrium or ovary. This, in fact, was secondary to carcinoma of the endometrium.

58 (a) Hypertropy of the gums with epulis of pregnancy.
(b) Bleeding as a consequence of trauma.
(d) An epulis of pregnancy typically regresses spontaneously after delivery.
(d) No.

59 (a) Pyogenic arthritis which, in this case, was gonococcal.
(b) Ankle, wrist and small joints of the hands, shoulder, hip or elbow.
(c) Aspiration of the joint fluid for culture.
(d) Blood culture and gonococcal compliment fixation tests may be positive. Urethral, cervical, rectal and pharyngeal swabs should be taken for culture from both the patient and her partner. Also check for other forms of sexually transmitted disease.

60 (a) Turner's syndrome.
(b) Sexual infantilism, short stature, primary amenorrhoea, webbing of the neck, wide carrying angle of the arms and shield-shaped chest.
(c) Coarctation of the aorta and congenital abnormalities of the renal collecting system.
(d) Yes, mosaics may occur and, therefore, karyotyping should be done because the management or prognosis for fertility may be modified.

61 (a) Diabetes mellitus.

(b) Treatment should include scrupulous control of blood sugars by serial blood sugar profiles, careful dietary regulation and administration of insulin as required.

(c) Hypoglycaemia, hypocalcaemia, hypomagnesaemia, polycythaemia, hyper bilirubinaemia, jaundice, birth trauma, respiratory distress syndrome and macrosomia. The incidence of congenital abnormality is also increased.

(d) No, but there may be a strong family history.

62 *Top*—Simpson's forceps (similar to Neville Barnes without axis traction)
Below—Kielland's forceps.

(b) Kielland's forceps have a sliding lock, longer shanks and minimal pelvic curve.

(c) Rotation from occipito-transverse or occipito-posterior (mid- or low cavity) as the minimal pelvic curve minimises maternal trauma in rotation, the long shanks compensate for loss of station in rotation, and the sliding lock allows for a degree of asynclitism.

(d) For the head arrested high and transverse, unengaged or just engaging. High forceps deliveries are no longer acceptable in modern obstetrical practice.

63 (a) The upper limbs are short and the femora are 'telephone shaped'.

(b) The skull is sclerotic, the vertebrae are 'H-shaped' and the ribs are short and club-ended.

(c) Thanatophoric (death-seeking) Dwarfism.

(d) In view of the hard skull, moulding does not occur and cephalic disproportion may arise.

64 (a) A succenturiate lobe.

(b) No.

(c) As a vasa praevia.

(d) Retained products of conception resulting in postpartum haemorrhage.

65 (a) Urethral caruncle, prolapsed urethral mucosa or carcinoma.

(b) Examination under anaesthesia and excision for histology.

(c) Prolapsed urethral mucosa with thrombosis (similar to haemorrhoids).

(d) No.

66,67 (a) Yes.

(b) Most patients, but not all, are found to have concurrent amoebiasis.

(c) Painful.

(d) Yes.

68 (a) Leiomyomata, fibromata, lipomata, neurofibromata or neuro-lemmomata (nerve sheath tumour).

(b) Fibromata and leiomyomata.

(c) Yes, with larger tumours.

(d) Yes, because secondary infection is also common.

69 (a) There is vaginal wall prolapse with ulceration but the components of the prolapse are difficult to identify from the photograph.

(b) 80 to 90 per cent.

(c) No.

(d) Almost certainly, in order to obtain a cure in the majority of cases.

70 (a) Adenomyosis and small fibroids.

(b) Between 35 and 45 years.

(c) Menorrhagia and dysmenorrhoea.

(d) An enlarged uterus, probably about twice normal size.

1 (a) Two endometrial glands with some cells showing subnuclear vacuolation.

(b) Dilatation and curettage or outpatient endometrial aspiration biopsy (Vabra).

(c) Mid-cycle. The endometrium is in transition from proliferative to secretory phase.

(d) It indicates that ovulation probably has occurred.

2 (a) Ligate the cord as close to the placenta as possible or at the cervix and leave the placenta *in situ*.

(b) No.

(c) About 2 years.

(d) Placenta increta where the placenta penetrates the uterine muscle and placenta percreta where penetration has reached the peritoneal surface of the uterus.

3 (a) Double (bicornuate bicollis) uterus.

(b) There are small fimbrial cysts visible at each fundus.

(c) There is an increased incidence of breech presentation.

(d) Premature labour and an increased incidence of operative delivery.

4 (a) Probably nothing since one has either cured the patient or, if there is spread outside the uterus, it is beyond control.

(b) No, although there are haemorrhagic areas present.

(c) Possibly less than 0.5 per cent.

(d) No, as malignant change is uncommon and especially as patients now tend to present at an earlier age with fibroids.

5 (a) 'Lump down below', dragging sensation, backache, with urinary symptoms or, possibly, difficulty with defaecation and bleeding.

(b) Congenital laxity of tissues, postmenopausal atrophy, obstetric history of difficult labours or deliveries, obesity or chronic chest symptoms.

(c) Surgical, either a repair operation and vaginal hysterectomy or a Manchester repair operation.

(d) Insertion of a pessary either as a temporary measure or as treatment if the patient is unfit for operation.

6 (a) Membranes are visible at a partially open cervical os.

(b) Incompetent cervix.

(c) Weakness or deficiency of the cervical fibro-muscular tissue and either congenital or acquired, eg manual dilatation of the cervix to more than 8 mm, cone biopsy or cervical amputation.

(d) Cervical circlage with a non-absorbable suture early in the second trimester. Attempts should be made to place the suture as near to the internal os as possible.

7 (a) 50 years, for the cervix is smaller than expected for a patient aged 30 years.

(b) An IVP because the staging would be III if there were hydronephrosis or hydroureter.

(c) Not if the diagnosis had already been made histologically.

(d) Squamous cell carcinoma.

8 (a) Repeated vaginal surgical attempts to correct her urinary symptoms.

(b) Scarring has destroyed the sphincteric mechanism and is effectively holding the urethra open.

(c) Urethral reconstruction or formation of a neourethra, use of an artificial sphincter or urinary diversion.

(d) Genuine stress incontinence (urethral sphincter incontinence); destrusc instability either primary or secondary to a neuropathic disorder; retentio with overflow; congenital abnormalities; fistulae; functional disorders.

79 (a) The presence of a vaginal septum with two speculae inserted. Th cervix is exposed on the left side.
(b) Renal tract abnormalities, which is the reason for always doing an IVP o such patients.
(c) With the usual measures, including analgesics and antispasmodics. In thi patient neither these nor dilatation of the cervices helped. The only relief wa obtained by oral contraceptive therapy.
(d) Sometimes none, but abortion, malpresentations and premature labou are recognised complications of uterine abnormalities when these are presen in association with the septum. The septum may cause obstruction in labou and require removal.

80 (a) Fallopian tube overlying portion of ovary and, on the right of th picture, bowel is seen.
(b) Hydrotubation with methylene blue dye to demonstrate tubal patency.
(c) Yes, but complete assessment requires observation of spill of dye from th fimbrial end of the tube.
(d) Anaesthetic, embolic, infection, haemorrhage, perforation of variou organs and structures.

81 (a) Torsion.
(b) Yes, but only in rare circumstances. In the majority of cases the treatmen will be by salpingo-oophorectomy.
(c) Rupture, haemorrhage or malignant change.
(d) Pain.

82 (a) An enlarged pituitary fossa.
(b) Prolactin.
(c) Amenorrhoea, galactorrhoea and symptoms of deficient oestrogenisatio such as vaginal dryness.
(d) Check the visual fields and assess for evidence of inappropriate secretio of other pituitary hormones which sometimes occurs. The X-ray is from a acromegalic patient.

83 (a) Intermenstrual discharge or bleeding and possibly pain.
(b) Pre-menopausal or within the reproductive age group, as one ovary a least was conserved.
(c) A necrotic uterine polyp.
(d) No.

84 (a) A lateral cystogram showing contrast medium leaking through a vesic or high urethral fistula.
(b) Operative and obstetric trauma, radiotherapy, ulceration secondary foreign bodies or chemicals in the vagina.
(c) Fistulas in the distal urethra may leak only during micturition and th patient complains of dribbling urine (from the vagina where it has poole after voiding. More proximal urethral and vesico-vaginal fistulas will lea continuously.
(d) No.

85 (a) Chloasma with butterfly-shaped distribution of pigmentation.
(b) Use of the combined oestrogen/progestogen oral contraceptive pill.
(c) Marked linea nigra, and pigmentation of the areola of the nipples.
(d) If pregnant, no. If caused by the pill, it does not usually regress com pletely.

6 (a) In certain cultures, notably in the Papua New Guinea highlands, it is traditional to amputate terminal phalanges on the death of a child or male relative.

b) Two.

c) Female circumcision in Africa, which is still performed although it is now illegal everywhere. Apart from mutilation, the urethra may become hidden by a bridge of skin and deflect the urinary stream. The continual splashing of the thighs may be followed by chronic infection of the constantly wet skin.

7 (a) Monilial (candida) vulvo-vaginitis treated by Nystatin (or similar topical or anti-fungal agents).

b) Broad spectrum antibiotics, diabetes mellitus, oral contraceptive therapy, pregnancy or immunosuppression.

c) Vulval dystrophy. The vaginal orifice is gaping, suggesting that a cystocele might be present.

d) For vulval dystrophy—eradication of infection, advice on vulval hygiene, application of topical steroids and regular review. Often multiple biopsies will be necessary to confirm the diagnosis and exclude preinvasive and invasive disease. For a vaginal wall prolapse—depending upon the symptoms remaining after treatment of the infection, anterior colporrhaphy may be required.

8,89 (a) Metastatic carcinoma in the umbilicus—'Sister Joseph's nodule.

b) Secondary carcinoma, hernia, endometriosis or lipoma.

c) Via the lymphatics of the obliterated hypogastric artery and urachus.

d) Visceral and parietal peritoneum, omentum and para-aortic nodes.

0 (a) From the left, a shelf pessary, a Hodge pessary and a ring pessary.

b) In general, the shelf and ring pessary may be used for the non-operative treatment of uterovaginal prolapse, either as a temporary measure (in those awaiting surgery or pregnant patients) or as a long-term treatment (in the elderly or those unfit for surgery). The Hodge pessary may be used for a trial period to antevert a retroverted uterus to which symptoms such as dyspareunia are attributed.

c) Ulcerated vaginal epithelium in the elderly.

d) By changing the pessary every 4–6 months in association with a course of topical oestrogen cream, eg dienoestrol.

1 (a) It occurs in a proportion of pregnant women as a consequence of their elevated circulatory oestrogen levels. Presumably, in these women their liver is less able to cope with the metabolism of the increased oestrogen.

b) Spider naevi.

c) The fetal alcohol syndrome is well recognised and is characterised by craniofacial, limb and cardiovascular defects as well as prenatal and postnatal growth deficiency and developmental delay.

d) An elevated MCV and raised hepatic enzymes, notably gamma glutamyl transferase.

2 (a) Carcinoma of the cervix.

b) That she has an early cancer which can be cured with early treatment but it depends upon what she and her husband wish in relation to the pregnancy. If the lesion is Stage IB or early IIA, then a radical hysterectomy with ovarian conservation and pelvic lymphadenectomy is the preferred treatment in a patient of this age and gestation. If the couple wish to continue with the pregnancy, then the patient should be delivered by Caesarean section as soon as the baby is considered viable.

c) Ensure that the patient is delivered in a hospital with adequate neonatal resources. Plan for delivery at 30–32 weeks giving steroid, (eg dexa-

methasone, weekly from the 28th week) to mature the fetal lungs. After delivery, a radical hysterectomy and pelvic lymphadenectomy or radio therapy could be the treatment depending upon individual preference, experience and facilities.
(d) If treated immediately, probably 80-90 per cent have 5-year survival.

93 (a) Clitoral hypertrophy; note the shaven pubic region.
(b) Congenital deficiency in enzymes necessary for conversion of pregnenolone to cortisol. Most frequently C-21 hydroxylase, less frequently C-1 alpha hydroxylase or C-11 hydroxylase and least frequently 3 beta hydroxysteroid dehydrogenase deficiency. 5-alpha reductase deficiency is a further possibilty.
(c) If the problem is the adrenogenital syndrome, then the phenotype will be female, the gonads will be ovaries and the chromosomal pattern 46 XX. If 5-alpha reductase deficiency is present, then the phenotype will be female the gonads testes and the chromosomal pattern 46 XY.
(d) With corticosteroids and local corrective surgery for the adrenogenital syndrome. With 5-alpha reductase deficiency, the gonads should be removed and corrective surgery may also be required.

94 (a) Obstructed labour.
(b) Delay in dilatation and descent. Meconium staining of liquor indicating possible fetal distress.
(c) Presence of maternal tachycardia, haematuria and the development of a uterine retraction ring (Bandl's ring).
(d) An apparent large fetal size, the presentation and position of the fetus descent of the presenting part as assessed upon abdominal examination and increased caput and moulding. A change in the fetal heart rate pattern may also be important.

95 (a) Transverse lie, with the back down and the head on the left.
(b) Uterine abnormality, placenta praevia, pelvic tumour, high parity, prematurity, multiple pregnancy, contracted pelvis, fetal death in utero or poly hydramnios.
(c) There is no obvious skeletal abnormality visible.
(d) Approximately 25 per cent.

96 (a) Loss of short, and long-term variability.
(b) Short-term variability is reduced early in fetal hypoxia; drugs which depress the central nervous system or autonomic responses.
(c) There is normally a gradual increase in fetal heart rate variablity as gestational age advances.
(d) No.

97 (a) Second trimester.
(b) It is even more difficult than the usual tubal pregnancy.
(c) This is not usually a consideration because of the poor clinical condition o the patient.
(d) In very rare circumstances the pregnancy reimplants and an extrauterine pregnancy continues.

98 (a) Sarcoma botryoides.
(b) The presence of local, regional or disseminated disease. Operative resectability, lymph node involvement and microscopic residual disease.
(c) Yes. Formerly, pelvic exenteration with pelvic wall node dissection and vulvectomy was used; now surgery, less extensive than exenteration, is followed by combined chemotherapy.
(d) Bloody discharge, vaginal bleeding and a mass.

(a) A malignant melanoma.
) Radical vulvectomy and regional lymphadenectomy.
) Various studies suggest 3–9 per cent.
) In general, poor.

0 (a) Yes.
) Haemophilus ducreyi.
) Yes and bubo formation in regional nodes occurs in about 50 per cent of omen.
) Erythromycin 500 mg, 6-hourly for 10 days and until the ulcers and lymph des have healed. Tetracycline and sulphadiazine may also be used.

1,102 (a) Ritual circumcision.
) Either difficulty with intercourse or with micturition.
Incision of the tissue covering the middle finger until the urethra is vealed and exposed.
) No, it is not usually affected.

3 (a) Hysterectomy with midline uterine incision.
) The most probable reason would be cervical malignancy in pregnancy. e cuff of vagina supports this. Hysterectomy may be required also for controlled bleeding, following classical Caesarian section.
Colposcopy and cervical biopsy. Wedge or cone biopsy may be needed for definitive diagnosis but cone biopsy is usually avoided in pregnancy.
) Dangers from premature delivery, rather than the cervical disease.

4 (a) Normal.
) Mature and immature.
) Yes; no.

5 (a) A decidual cast.
) Ectopic pregnancy.
) A gestation sac.
) On withdrawal of high levels of endogenous or exogenous progestogen.

6 (a) Hydatidiform mole.
) 40 years or over, but premenopausal.
) By the passage of vesicles per vagina.
) About 16–18 weeks.

7 (a) Ectopic gestation.
) Not since *in vitro* fertilisation has been introduced. It was suggested that the presence of an ectopic pregnancy on one side and a corpus luteum on e other, ipsilateral oophorectomy may improve the subsequent pregnancy te.
) Cornual pregnancy; ovarian pregnancy; cervical pregnancy; pregnancy in rudimentary uterine horn or abdominal pregnancy.
) Abdominal pregnancy as a consequence of implantation after tubal apture, although this is very rare.

08 (a) It is probably secondary. It usually spreads from a pulmonary source the Fallopian tubes by a haematogenous route. Direct extension to other arts of the genital tract, including the cervix, may then occur.
) There is usually either an ulcerative lesion that can resemble cervical arcinoma, or a papillomatous lesion.
) Only 10–25 per cent.
) Although very rare this has been reported.

09 (a) 6–7 o'clock.
) A cone biopsy to confirm the diagnosis and assess the extent of the lesion, ther than proceed to a hysterectomy.

(c) This depends upon the staging of the tumour. For Stage IB lesions, th treatment of choice would be radical hysterectomy and pelvic lym phadenectomy with ovarian conservation. An alternative would be radio radiotherapy and, indeed, the facilities available may influence the metho of treatment.

(d) Conservative or radical treatment, either surgically or with radiotheraj is the choice. Tumour volume, extent and location are the primary factors be considered but in selected cases, conservative care with preservation fertility may be possible.

110 (a) The lesion is a syphilitic chancre.
(b) About 40 per cent.
(c) Yes, especially when hypertrophic.
(d) Yes, VDRL and FTA or other serological tests should be performed an if negative, repeated in 4 weeks. The fetus may be infected from placent spread resulting in an infant with congenital syphilis or a late stillbirth.

111 (a) Metastatic lesion from an endometrial carcinoma.
(b) Radiotherapy.
(c) Lymphatic or vascular.
(d) Although adjuvant radiotherapy will reduce the incidence of metastat lesions in the lower genital tract, it will not entirely prevent them even given to the whole length of the vagina.

112 (a) Inflammatory cells.
(b) Cervicitis secondary to infection.
(c) Gonorrhoea, Chlamydia and puerperal infection.
(d) Herpes, syphilis or chancroid.

113 (a) The urethra has been opened longitudinally to show both internal ar external meatuses. The anterior vaginal wall has been incised beyond this.
(b) Urinary incontinence caused by a urethral fistula following anterii colporrhaphy.
(c) Repair in two or three layers with catgut or polyglycolic acid sutures ov a splint. Non-absorbable sutures may be used but should be removed later.
(d) Continuous suprapubic drainage for 10–12 days or vaginal cystostomy.

114 (a) Paroxysmal attacks of hypertension, headache, sweating, elevation body temperature, abdominal pain or palpitations but there would be r proteinuria.
(b) In the adrenal medulla.
(c) Yes. Sometimes after the removal of the phaeochromocytoma loc recurrence and metastases develop.
(d) The levels of catecholamines (adrenaline and noradrenaline) are raise The measurement of VMA (vanilmandelic acid) or of HMMA (3-methoxy-hydroxymandelic acid) excretion in urine is also diagnostic.

115 (a) A least Stage III because there is evidence of hydronephrosis, espec ally on the left.
(b) In patients with recurrent disease after previous treatment, to asse operability when exenteration is being considered.
(c) Directed fine needle aspiration cytology.
(d) Ovarian tumours, to assess the effectiveness of chemotherapy.

116 (a) Ovarian cystectomy.
(b) If it looks normal, no.
(c) Yes, there is nothing to be lost by taking a specimen.
(d) It is debatable but there is probably no justification for the procedure.

17 (a) There is a large calcified pelvic mass with a second smaller calcified mass adjacent. No fractures are evident.
(b) A calcified fibroid.
(c) Check pelvic findings and, if consistent with a fibroid uterus, then no treatment would be required apart from clinical review, if the patient were asymptomatic. Progressive increase in size of the tumour would demand surgical intervention.
(d) Torsion of the fibroid, if subserous. Sarcomatous degeneration, although this is very rare.

18 (a) Liquid (usually water or 0.9 per cent saline) at body temperature or gas (carbon dioxide).
(b) Inappropriate temperature or very fast filling are non-physiological and may provoke detrusor activity. Gas may irritate the bladder mucosa and there are difficulties in estimating leakage and measuring the voiding rate and residual volumes.
(c) General physical examination, cystourethroscopy, uroflowmetry, urethral pressure measurements and electromyography.
(d) No, normal detrusor pressure on filling is less than 15cm H_2O.

19 (a) Bladder distension.
(b) By catheterisation.
(c) It may be prevented from descending into the pelvis and therefore remain high and mobile.
(d) No, the appearance is different.

20 (a) Subconjunctival haemorrhage.
(b) 'Pushing' in second stage of labour.
(c) Petechial haemorrhages in the skin of head, neck and shoulders.
(d) None.

21 (a) Rare fibromata which occur in pregnancy (molluscum fibrosum gravidarum).
(b) They result from simple epithelial hyperplasia.
(c) Pedunculated lesions can be dealt with by ligating the base; sessile lesions can be cauterised or excised.
(d) Upper chest.

22 (a) Iron deficiency anaemia.
(b) The conjunctivae, nails, hands and palmar creases.
(c) A microcytic, hypochromic anaemia.
(d) In the first instance, the patient would need blood transfusion by the slow administration of packed red blood cells and possibly the administration of diuretics. If there were cardiovascular compromise then exchange transfusions may be used. Restoration of iron stores and treatment of the menorrhagia would subsequently be required.

23 (a) An ovarian cyst.
(b) Dullness of percussion and shifting dullness if ascites present.
(c) An ultrasonic scan.
(d) Assess whether the mass appears malignant by inspection of the pelvic organs, pelvic peritoneum, paracolic gutters, surface of the diaphragm, omentum and para-aortic nodes. Samples of any free fluid or peritoneal washings should be taken. A total abdominal hysterectomy and bilateral salpingo-oophorectomy should then be performed and if malignancy is suspected an omentectomy should be included.

24 (a) Coronal suture, frontal bones with frontal suture, anterior fontanelle (bregma), temporal bone, occipital bone, lambdoid suture, supra-orbital ridge, orbit, nasion, parietal eminence and the frontal eminence (mentum).

(b) Biparetal diameter 9.5 cm; suboccipitobregmatic 9.5 cm.
(c) In a face presentation the fetal head is fully extended, presenting th
submentobregmatic diameter which, however, has the same measurement a
the suboccipitobregmatic diameter.
(d) Moderate moulding is a physiological phenomenon which facilitates pro
gress in labour. Excessive moulding with marked overlap of cranial bones
evidence of significant disproportion.

125 (a) Brow.
(b) Mentovertical, the longest cranial diameter.
(c) Anterior fontanelle and supra-orbital ridges.
(d) Caesarean section. Vaginal delivery may occasionally be achieved in th
event of flexion to a vertex presentation, or deflexion to a mentoanterior fac
presentation.

126 (a) Late decelerations and baseline tachycardia.
(b) Onset of decelerations usually occurs 30 seconds or more after onset c
contraction, nadir occurs well after the contraction peak and returns t
baseline after the contraction is over.
(c) Fetal hypoxia from compromised uteroplacental blood flow.
(d) Acidosis results in myocardial depression.

127,128 (a) Velamentous insertion of the cord.
(b) Vasa previa—fetal hypoxia if vascular compression, fetal exsanguinatio
if vascular rupture.
(c) The vessels may be palpated on vaginal examination (pulsating at feta
heart rate). There may also be intrapartum haemorrhage after rupture of th
membranes and signs of fetal distress (including a sinusoidal cardiotocograp
trace).
(d) It is possible to distinguish between blood from the mother and her fetu
because alkali denaturation of the blood will indicate fetal haemoglobin. Th
test is known as Apt's or Singer's test.

129 (a) Haematocolpos.
(b) Normal 46 XX.
(c) Incision of the membrane and allow natural drainage.
(d) No.

130 (a) In essence abnormal androgenic stimulation in utero, either over
stimulation of the female or understimulation of the male.
(b) Synthetic progestogens especially the 19 nortestosterone derivatives.
(c) Any newborn infant with ambiguity of the genitalia so marked that th
urethral opening is in the perineal area should be considered female.
(d) Never, cytogenetics from leukocyte culture should always be performed
Buccal smears were used in the past and were said to be reliable after tw
weeks.

131,132 (a) Paget's disease of the vulva-adenocarcinoma *in situ*.
(b) It is confined to the apocrine (sweat) gland region of the vulva.
(c) One third have an underlying sweat gland carcinoma–25 per cent have a
associated or prior malignancy elsewhere.
(d) Hyperchromatic nuclei and vacuolated cytoplasm.

133 (a) Probably reflects the previous application of a band in the hope tha
the tumour would slough away.
(b) Only partially.
(c) It became too painful.
(d) If excised properly at the base, no.

134 (a) Yes.

) This is always a debatable issue in which the patient and her husband ced to be involved. The options are for termination of the pregnancy and idical hysterectomy, or early delivery of a viable gestation followed by idical hysterectomy.

:) This depends upon the paediatric resources available. If facilities are ptimal, then delivery between 32-34 weeks could be contemplated. If mited, then 34-36 weeks.

1) In experienced hands there is no significant increase in morbidity. The rocedure may be therapeutic in the presence of early node metastases or rognostic in the sense that radiotherapy or chemotherapy may be indicated.

35 (a) A Dalkon shield (note the encrustations on the thread).

) A reported high incidence of ascending genital tract infection.

:) The device was manufactured with a woven multifilament rather than a 1onofilament thread, and this was thought to be associated with ascent of 1fection.

1) Pregnancy, past or present pelvic inflammatory disease, congenital or cquired deformity of the uterine cavity, valvular heart disease and con-itions in which infection is a problem such as a hip replacement, and 1bnormal genital tract bleeding until investigated. Allergy to materials in the evice would also be a contraindication.

36 (a) Cervical intraepithelial neoplasia grade I, with wart virus change.

) The transformation zone, that is the area of the cervix that was originally overed by columnar epithelium, but has subsequently been replaced with juamous epithelium by a process of metaplasia.

:) The patient usually presents with an abnormal Papanicolau smear.

1) Onset of sexual activity at an early age and multiple sexual partners are 1ajor risk factors.

37 (a) Bartholin's abscess.

) Neisseria gonorrhoeae.

:) With vaginal discharge, pelvic inflammatory disease, infertility, arthritis r a rash.

1) Marsupialisation and antibiotics if appropriate.

38 (a) Usually diagnosed late and mistaken for an ovarian tumour. The atient may have serous or sanguineous discharge (often described as watery), 1bdominal pain or a palpable mass.

) Commonly 45–60 years (50 per cent nulliparous) but certainly more ommon after the menopause.

:) Usually total hysterectomy with bilateral salpingo-oophorectomy fol-owed by radiotherapy or chemotherapy. Prognosis is poor.

1) 0.3 per cent of all gynaecological malignancies.

39 (a) They were subserous fibroids.

b) Hysterectomy would prevent further fibroid development, but it is not trictly necessary in a patient who is symptomless and the body of the uterus id not contain any other fibroids. It would also depend upon the patient's esire for pregnancy.

c) Opening the cavity is probably best avoided. It is preferable for a cur-ttage to be performed to exclude submucous fibroids.

d) This obviously varies with the type of ovarian tumour but as the peak age 1cidence for ovarian malignancy is 40–60 years, the risk of malignancy is robably at least 30 per cent. About a quarter of the deaths from ovarian ancer occur between 35 and 50 years. The figure usually quoted for sarcoma-ous change in fibroids is 0.5 per cent; however, the risk of malignancy in this ge group would be minimal.

140 (a) Endometriosis of the cervix.
(b) Pelvic peritoneum especially overlying the uterosacral ligaments, pouc of Douglas and ovarian fossae or the ovaries.
(c) As an incidental finding at laparoscopy or laparotomy, or in associatio with complaints of infertility, dysmenorrhoea, menorrhagia or dyspareunia.
(d) A high dose progesterone oral contraceptive pill for 6–9 months. Cor tinuous progesterone therapy (eg dydrogesterone). Danazol. LH–RH ana logues.

141 (a) Monilia (Candida albicans).
(b) Ideally, clear the vaginal infection with a topical anti-fungal agent such a Nystatin, prior to onset of labour. If the infection is still present at the time c delivery it may be advisable to treat the baby prophylactically.
(c) Diabetes mellitus, whether or not insulin dependent.
(d) A raw area which often bleeds.

142 (a) Gartner's duct cyst.
(b) Paraurethral cyst (Skene's duct cyst).
(c) By marsupialisation or excision of the cyst.
(d) Benign.

143 (a) Two small ulcers.
(b) Herpes cervicitis.
(c) Herpes hominis type II in 75–85 per cent of cases, although this pattern i changing to show a greater proportion of Herpes hominis type I.
(d) 3–7 days.

144 (a) A suburethral cyst.
(b) Benign.
(c) Marsupialisation of the cyst.
(d) No, very rarely infected.

145 (a) Yes, related to the menstrual cycle.
(b) Dyspareunia.
(c) With progestogens continuously, with an oestrogen/progestogen prepara tion continuously or with danazol for a period of 6–9 months.
(d) No, it would be better to add one of the above preparations for at least months.

146 (a) The entire epithelium has been replaced by atypical cells. There i loss of polarity and the cells appear crowded. Many cells have large darkly staining nuclei and there are numerous mitotic figures seen. These change are consistent with cervical intraepithelial neoplasia grade III.
(b) By colposcopy in association with cytological and histological assessment.
(c) If the lesion is visible in its entirety through the colposcope, there is n suspicion of invasion and the most colposcopically abnormal area has bee sampled histologically—then various methods of local ablative therapy ca be used. Laser vaporisation, electrocoagulation diathermy and cryotherap are all effective means of treatment. If these conditions are not fulfilled the a cone biopsy is necessary.
(d) The lesion can be observed with the aid of cytology, colposcopy an limited punch biopsies and treatment deferred until the postpartum period.

147 (a) Not unless there is a high index of suspicion.
(b) A chemical determination of the total pressor amines in the blood (adrer aline and noradrenaline).
(c) Yes.
(d) Possibly 1:3.

48,149 (a) The bladder.
b) No, there is an indentation on the right lower aspect.
c) Yes, on the right side there is a discrete enlarged lymph node.
d) No.

50 (a) Lateral micturating cystogram showing a urethral diverticulum.
b) Congenital, rupture of a periurethral abscess into the urethra, and surgical or obstetric trauma.
c) It may present as a local swelling, discomfort, dysuria, dyspareunia and dribbling of urine. The treatment is excision and closure of the urethral defect.
d) A calculus may be present and visible on X-ray.

51 (a) Suprapubic collateral circulation.
b) Deep vein thrombosis in the pelvis.
c) Pregnancy, the oral contraceptive pill, immobilisation, hypercoagulation and tumours.
d) Paramedian or midline thus avoiding a Pfannensteil incision which is likely to be associated with more bleeding.

52 (a) Cushing's syndrome.
b) A dexamethasone suppression test.
c) After the administration of dexamethasone at night, a morning cortisol level greater than 20 μg/100 dl signifies Cushing's syndrome. Intermediate values are indeterminant.
d) Yes, if the cause of Cushing's syndrome is determined and treated appropriately.

53 (a) A diathermy burn.
b) By proper application of the diathermy pad and routine checks on insulation.
c) Bipolar.
d) High frequency.

54 (a) Acromegaly.
b) With amenorrhoea. Ovulation is suppressed by associated hyperprolactinaemia or by reduced gonadotrophin production secondary to the pressure effects of the tumour.
c) By estimation of growth hormone (GH) but cross reaction with human placental lactogen may occur. The elevated levels of GH are not suppressed by a glucose load.
d) Pregnancy is rare even in the treated case, but when it occurs it is usually normal, producing an appropriately grown infant.

55 (a) There is an increase in factors I, II, VII, VIII, IX, X; a decrease in activity of the fibrinolytic system and reduced antithrombin III.
(b) Venous stasis, bed rest, age 35+ and parity, obesity and blood group A, AB or B and sickle cell disease. Any operative delivery and if oestrogen is given to suppress lactation.
(c) Warfarin results in a low but definite incidence of teratogenesis, most commonly chondrodysplasia punctata. In late pregnancy the risk is of retroplacental or fetal intracerebral haemorrhage. Heparin does not cross the placenta due to its high molecular weight and, therefore, does not pose a risk to the fetus.
(d) Bleeding, paradoxical intravascular thrombosis and haemorrhage (a plasma heparin dependent platelet aggregating factor results in platelet consumption and severe thrombocytopenia) and osteoporosis.

156,157 (a) Rounded inlet, straight walls, non-prominent spines, wide subpubic arch, rounded wide sacrosciatic notches and curved sacrum.
(b) Approximately 50 per cent.
(c) Triangular inlet, convergent side walls with prominent ischial spines narrow subpubic arch and narrow, high arched sacrosciatic notches and flat sacrum angled forward.
(d) Breech presentation, previous Caesarean section (where vaginal delivery is contemplated) and pelvic injury (especially road traffic accident). The use of pelvimetry for a cephalic presentation with suspected disproportion is controversial.

158 (a) Twin pregnancy, both twins presenting by the vertex.
(b) Increased anaemia, hyperemesis, varicose veins, haemorrhoids and oedema. Premature labour, premature rupture of membranes, antepartum haemorrhage, polyhydramnios, pre-eclampsia, intrauterine growth retardation, malpresentation, increased operative/manipulative deliveries, postpartum haemorrhage and increased perinatal mortality.
(c) Uniovular—one chorion, two amnions. Binovular—two chorions, two amnions.
(d) Before 38th week of gestation.

159 (a) A twin placenta with an umbilical cord on the left compatible with a viable fetus. The cord on the right is withered.
(b) Fetus papyraceous.
(c) No.
(d) Fetal death in utero of one twin. The retained dead fetus remains in utero as the living fetus continues to develop.

160 (a) Ventouse vacuum extraction.
(b) As for any operative delivery; soft tissue injury, bony injury or intracranial damage but, in the majority of cases there are no complications.
(c) Delay in the second stage of labour or for fetal distress. It is also useful to expedite delivery of a second twin, or when delivery is indicated in the presence of a small remaining rim, or lip, of the cervix.
(d) Empty bladder, rectum, presence of uterine contractions, reasonable chance of success, suitable presentation, membranes ruptured and preferably, full dilatation of the cervix.

161 (a) As the patient is likely to be elderly, the genital prolapse can be treated by reduction and insertion of a pessary. The rectal prolapse can only be treated conservatively by reduction.
(b) The vaginal pessary may be successful but the rectal prolapse will almost certainly recur.
(c) The vaginal prolapse appears to have been present for some time. The rectal prolapse is probably of recent onset.
(d) The rectal prolapse would require an abdominal operation, for support of the bowel. There are various techniques for this or alternatively a Thiersch wire could be used. Vaginal hysterectomy and repair, Manchester repair operation or colpocleisis are options for the genital prolapse.

162 (a) This is a typical vulvitis in a diabetic, the organism involved usually being fungal.
(b) Diabetic control, vulval hygiene and anti-fungal preparations as necessary.
(c) On these appearances, no.
(d) No, it would be totally unjustified.

163 (a) Basal cell carcinoma (rodent ulcer).
(b) Biopsy and histology.
(c) Local excision.
(d) Face.

164 (a) A scaly lesion characterised by a red background dotted with white hyperkeratotic islands as shown.
(b) A common complaint is that of pruritus but it could present as a lump or be relatively asymptomatic.
(c) There is loss of normally layered architecture with full thickness replacement by atypical juvenile cells. Features of acanthosis and hyperkeratosis and parakeratosis may be seen.
(d) No, the correct term is vulval intraepithelial neoplasia, Grade III (VIN III).

165 (a) The taking of a vulval smear and clinical follow-up.
(b) No.
(c) Hypotrophic.
(d) No.

166 (a) Probably premenopausal as an ovary has been conserved.
(b) Pain or discomfort due to a fibroid prolapsing through the cervix.
(c) The ureters would be particularly at risk due to the expanded size of the cervix.
(d) A submucus leiomyoma of the uterus.

167 (a) Material obtained probably represented old altered pus.
(b) It is probably a dermoid cyst as there appears to be a tooth present at about 3 o'clock.
(c) Yes, if a dermoid or tubo-ovarian pyosalpinx.
(d) The reproductive age group, particularly 20–35 years.

168 (a) Postmenopausal because ovarian tumours are more common in this age group.
(b) Vertical incision either midline or paramedian to allow adequate access of the upper and lower abdomen for removal and proper staging.
(c) Check for free fluid (ascites) and take peritoneal washings. Inspect the peritoneum, omentum, liver, diaphragm, and para-aortic nodes after initial assessment of the pelvic organs. Because of the likelihood of malignancy, proper staging should be done.
(d) Front as there is a portion of the left round ligament present and the ovarian ligament on the left side is not visible.

169 (a) Normal female breasts plus hirsutism.
(b) Constitutional hirsutism, polycystic ovarian disease, adrenal hyperplasia or overactivity and, rarely, a masculinising tumour of the ovary.
(c) Blood testosterone, androstenedione, sex hormone binding globulin, cortisol, and the LH:FSH ratio.
(d) Cyproterone acetate.

170 (a) Herpes.
(b) By culture and isolation of the virus.
(c) Until they re-epithelialise.
(d) Yes, but more usually with symptomatic lesions.

171 (a) A Lippes loop intrauterine contraceptive device on the right side of the pelvis.
(b) Pelvic ultrasound (X-ray with uterine sound *in situ* may be helpful in the absence of ultrasound facilities). Dilatation and curettage, hysteroscopy or laparoscopy. In rare cirumstances translocation into the bladder has been

reported and cystoscopy may be indicated.
(c) Removal by laparoscopy or laparotomy if an extrauterine site is confirmed.
(d) Oral contraception or barrier methods.

172 (a) Unicornuate uterus without filling of Fallopian tube.
(b) Yes, IVP.
(c) Absent right kidney.
(d) Both ovaries and the left Fallopian tube should be present. The right tube would be absent because of failure of development on this side.

173 (a) A colposcope.
(b) To take photographs for recording the findings during examination.
(c) Teaching purposes so that the colposcopist can demonstrate the findings while still using the bifocal eyepieces.
(d) It allows abnormal areas to be biopsied under direct vision which, combined with local ablative therapy, reduces the number of cone biopsies required.

174,175 (a) No, not without histological knowledge of the gonads.
(b) Yes, especially on the left side.
(c) From the illustrations, it is impossible to tell; they could be any combination but at least one is likely to be an ovotestis.
(d) Yes.

176 (a) Yes.
(b) No.
(c) Yes.
(d) Yes.

177 (a) Fetal tachycardia as evidenced by a baseline of 210 beats per minute (normal range 110–160).
(b) Pyrexia or hyperthyroidism.
(c) Hypoxia, anaemia, cardiac failure, tachyarrythmia or chorioamnionitis.
(d) Parasympathetic drugs (eg atropine), phenothiazines and beta sympathomimetic drugs (eg salbutamol, ritodrine).

178 (a) Hydatidiform mole.
(b) 80 per cent of patients with hydatidiform mole experience normal uterine involution and resumption of normal menstrual cycles without malignant sequelae.
(c) A large uterus, bilateral ovarian enlargement, maternal age greater than 40 years and past gestational trophoblastic disease.
(d) If still elevated after 10–12 weeks, by which time the majority have returned to normal.

179 (a) Gastroschisis, hare lip, abnormality of foot and hand.
(b) Separation of the amnion from the chorion with repair by mesoblastic proliferation.
(c) Digital constriction rings, craniofacial defects, syndactyly and club foot.
(d) No, careful inspection of the placental surface may be needed to find them.

180 (a) Intrauterine growth retardation of Twin 2. There may have been a relatively smaller proportion of the placenta available to this twin, or there may have been a placental arterio-venous shunt present.
(b) Possibly 5 to 6 times more common than uniovular.
(c) This depends upon the timing of division of the fertilised ovum but has ranged from 18 to 36 per cent in various reports.
(d) Race, maternal family history, maternal age, parity and drugs used for ovulation induction.

181 (a) Haematocolpos.
(b) A hydrocolpos.
(c) Yes.
(d) At an earlier age.

182 (a) Vulval dystrophy (Lichen sclerosis).
(b) Yes, the majority improve at the menarche.
(c) Topical hydrocortisone for symptomatic relief, but not as constant and prolonged therapy as it may produce atrophy and fibrosis in subepithelial tissue.
(d) About 2–3 per cent.

183 (a) Seborrhoeic eczema.
(b) Axillae, natal cleft and submammary region, umbilicus and skin folds in obese patients.
(c) No, but there may be secondary bacterial or fungal infection. Satellite lesions here suggest monilia infection.
(d) Keep the skin dry; treat specific infections; advise the patient to lose weight. Topical corticosteroid creams may be used.

184 (a) Probably by the application of topical corticosteroid preparations.
(b) Every 4–6 months for life, due to the chronic nature of the condition and possible development of malignancy.
(c) Vulval biopsies may be the only way to determine the development of malignancy, but there is contoversy over how often they should be done. If there is no change in symptoms then 2–3 yearly intervals may be reasonable.
(d) Benign hyperplastic.

185 (a) A pedunculated lipoma arising from the vulva.
(b) Usually as a lump or swelling that is often relatively symptomless.
(c) Ulceration and trauma.
(d) Surgical excision.

186 (a) No.
(b) If there had been no rupture of the ovarian capsule at the time of operation, then observation at regular intervals would be appropriate.
(c) Hormone replacement therapy would be contraindicated.
(d) Despite the previous Pfannensteil incision, it would be preferable to use a vertical incision because of the possiblity of adhesions and the possible presence of an ovarian tumour.

187 (a) A condylomatous plaque on the posterior lip of the cervix.
(b) Human papilloma virus.
(c) Cervical cytology, colposcopy and colposcopically directed biopsies, to exclude associated intraepithelial neoplasia.
(d) Regular follow-up and cytological assessment.

188,189 (a) Both show congenital abnormalities of the uterus. **188** is a completely duplicated system of the uterus, cervix and septate vagina, termed uterus didelphys. **189** demonstrates a double uterus with single cervix and vagina, termed bicornis unicollis.
(b) Fusion anomalies of the Mullerian (paramesonephric) duct systems.
(c) Tenth week.
(d) The woman with the bicornuate uterus (**189**). A septate, subseptate or bicornuate uterus may be implicated in recurrent abortion, antepartum haemorrhage, premature labour, malpresentation and retained placenta.

190 (a) No; there is a cervical ectopy present.
(b) Nothing.
(c) Ideally, within six months, after which routine cytology can be performed, if the next report is normal. This will minimise the risk of a false negative result when initiating cytology screening.

191 (a) Six weeks or later after the primary infection.
(b) Yes, generalised and non-tender lymphadenopathy.
(c) Yes.
(d) The infant may be stillborn, or may be liveborn but severely afflicted with congenital syphilis.

192 (a) It is characterised by dimpling of the skin and is caused by lymphatic oedema.
(b) There are stretch marks characteristic of pregnancy and it is therefore probable that this is associated with pre-eclampsia.
(c) Generalised oedema, albuminuria and hypertension.

193 (a) Gum hypertrophy.
(b) Phenytoin therapy and recently it has been noted with nifedipine.
(c) Increased incidence of congenital heart disease, cleft lip and palate, digital hypoplasia, haemolytic disease of the newborn. Syndrome of craniofacial and limb abnormalites, growth and mental retardation.
(d) Pregnancy.

194 (a) Condylomata lata of secondary syphilis.
(b) Very infective.
(c) Symmetrical maculopapular non-pruritic rash, often involving soles and palms. Mucous ulcers, non-tender lymphadenopathy, pharyngitis, nephritis, hepatosplenomegaly, iritis, conjunctivitis, periostitis, alopecia or low grade fever.
(d) All serological tests are positive at this stage. Treponema pallidium specific tests such as FTA-ABS are commonly used to confirm the diagnosis.

195 (a) The Cardiff 'count-to-ten' fetal activity chart.
(b) Starting at 9 o'clock in the morning, count the number of movements until the total equals 10, and record on the chart the half-hour during which this occurs. If less than 10 experienced, record the number in the lower section.
(c) Less than 10 movements for 2 days in a row or no movements in one day.
(d) Fetal heart auscultation and cardiotocography.

196 (a) A normal singleton fetus with cephalic presentation, and Lippes loop (IUCD), presumably *in situ* (a lateral view would be required to confirm).
(b) Spontaneous abortion or septic abortion.
(c) The placenta and membranes should be examined for the IUCD. If it were not found and the patient had an epidural for the conduct of her labour, then manual exploration of the uterus would be reasonable. Otherwise, an ultrasound scan or X-ray in the postpartum period could be used to locate the device.
(d) Assuming that the device had been intrauterine, then contraception would be entirely at the patient's request—the failure rate for the next IUCD would not be any higher.

197 (a) Sinusoidal pattern.
(b) It is considered an alarming sign of fetal distress.
(c) Severe fetal anaemia. It has also been reported after intrauterine intraperitoneal transfusion and related to the drug alphaprodine (a narcotic analgesic).
(d) (i) Immediate delivery by Caesarean section as this pattern implies impending fetal death unless the underlying anaemia is amenable to treatment in utero; (ii) take a fetal scalp pH as the prognosis of this pattern in labour is less certain.

198 (a) A Copper 7 intrauterine contraceptive device embedded in a placenta (see bottom of the photograph).
(b) 2–4 per 100 woman-years in the first year of use.
(c) Increased risk of spontaneous abortion, septic abortion, premature delivery, premature rupture of the membranes, stillbirth, ectopic pregnancy.
(d) After discussion with the patient an attempt should be made to remove the device if the tail is visible. If not, the device should be left *in situ*.

199 (a) Spina bifida.
(b) Hydrocephaly.
(c) Serum alpha fetoprotein, as a screening test. Amniotic fluid alpha fetoprotein, is a definitive test. Amniotic fluid acetylcholine esterase and detailed ultrasound scanning are also useful.
(d) Approximately 1:200.

200 (a) It is a haematoma usually caused by injury to the periosteum of the skull during labour and delivery.
(b) It can happen in the absence of birth trauma when haemostasis is defective.
(c) The swelling, which may be bilateral, usually overlies the parietal bones and is sharply limited to the area of the bone. This distinguishes the lesion from *caput succedaneum*.
(d) It may enlarge during the first 2 days of life (and may not be present for a few hours after delivery) and thereafter remains unchanged for 2–3 weeks. It then subsides slowly in subsequent months.

201 (a) Vulval haematoma.
(b) Falling astride a rigid fixed object, eg cross-bar of a bicycle, or falling on to a fence or metal bar.
(c) No.
(d) No.

202 (a) Vulval soreness and pruritus vulvae.
(b) 50–60 years or older.
(c) No. While relief of symptoms may be obtained, they tend to recur even if a vulvectomy is performed.
(d) Leukoplakia. This means a white patch of skin and has been applied to almost every 'white' lesion on the vulva. However, it is a non-specific term and should be avoided.

203 (a) Labial adhesions.
(b) After separation of the labia, regular application of oestrogen cream to prevent refusion.
(c) Yes, by regular application of local oestrogen cream, when the labia will often separate spontaneously after a week or two.
(d) Inflammation.

204 (a) Uterovaginal prolapse, at least second degree.
(b) Reduction of the prolapse with the aid of a pessary.
(c) Either a Manchester repair or a repair operation with vaginal hysterectomy.
(d) About 30 per cent.

205 (a) The peak incidence is in the 3rd and 4th decades.
(b) Usually quoted as 20–50 per cent.
(c) Various studies have suggested 30–45 per cent.
(d) Yes, in both instances papillary projections or processes.

206 (a) To remove cervical mucous and allow unstained cervical architecture to be studied.
(b) Yes, a clearer view of the capillaries is obtained if a green filter is used.
(c) Yes, a carcinoma has almost entirely replaced the cervix.
(d) Acetic acid (3 or 5 per cent) and any acetowhite area are considered abnormal. Iodine where unstained (relatively glycogen depleted) areas indicate regions of rapid cell growth and are abnormal.

207 (a) Vaginal septum.
(b) Coital difficulties, difficulty in using tampons or it may be an asymptomatic discovery at routine antenatal or gynaecological examination.
(c) A fetal head may slip past—if not, clamp divide and ligate. Breech may present astride and cause serious tearing.
(d) Double uterus and cervix, in which case also look for renal tract anomalies.

208 (a) Hysterosalpingography.
(b) Bilateral hydrosalpinges without any spill of the radio-opaque material.
(c) Laproscopy and direct visualisation of Fallopian tubes as assessment for tubal surgery or in-vitro fertilisation (IVF). Other potential causes for infertility, of necessity, would have to be evaluated.
(d) Tubal surgery of IVF.

209 (a) Tetracycline staining of the teeth.
(b) Yes, by the avoidance of maternal tetracycline therapy during pregnancy.
(c) No.
(d) Yes, preferably using local anaesthesia if an anaesthetic is required.

210 (a) Frank breech.
(b) External cephalic version.
(c) Antepartum haemorrhage, hypertension, pre-eclampsia, multiple pregnancy, uterine scar, threatened premature labour, and any absolute indication for Caesarean section. Certain fetal abnormalities are best managed as a breech, eg hydrocephalus.
(d) Check fetal heart rate and regularity. Kleihauer test and Anti-D in Rh negative women.

211 (a) A triplet placenta.
(b) 1:6,400.
(c) 1:3:2 (monozygotic:dizygotic:trizygotic)
(d) The predisposing factors are the same as for twins, namely advancing maternal age, increasing parity and maternal family history of multiple pregnancy. In particular, ovulation induction with gonadotrophins and ovarian hyperstimulation for in vitro fertilisation, with multiple embryo transfer are the most common predisposing factors.

212 (a) Immune hydrops has been reduced in incidence by the administration of anti-D gamma globulin to all non-immunised Rhesus negative women with Rhesus positive babies.
(b) Failure to administer anti-D gamma globulin to appropriate patients and antenatal sensitisation of the mother (where antenatal and anti-D gamma globulin is not given) are possible reasons for maternal immunisation. Occasionally, the dose of anti-D given is insufficient and the mother becomes sensitised. In addition there are various non-immunological causes for hydropic infants.
(c) Following the delivery of an infant with immunological hydrops, the next pregnancy is likely to be affected if the fetus is Rhesus positive. The disease tends to be more severe and develops at an earlier gestation in successive pregnancies.

(d) Cardiac anomalies, renal anomalies, gastrointestinal anomalies, chromosomal abnormalities, malformation syndromes, alpha thalassaemia, twin-to-twin transfusion syndrome, congenital infection and placental chorioangioma.

213 (a) Unusual facies, epicanthic folds, flattened nose and low set ears.
(b) Potter's syndrome. Renal agenesis.
(c) Intrauterine growth retardation, oligohydramnios, absent kidneys and lack of bladder filling on late pregnancy scan.
(d) Uniformly fatal. One third are stillborn, all others result in neonatal death, primarily due to pulmonary hypoplasia.

214 (a) Herpes simplex virus (HSV) Type 2.
(b) The cervix.
(c) Probably from active cervical lesions from where virus is shed into the genital tract.
(d) Symptomatic relief of symptoms plus acyclovir triphosphate therapy.

215 (a) Procidentia plus carcinoma of the vagina.
(b) Vaginal hysterectomy and repair in the first instance. Other factors such as the extent of the clearance and the age of the patient would determine whether postoperative therapy is given.
(c) Squamous cell carcinoma of the vagina.
(d) Pain or bleeding mainly; an offensive odour or discharge possibly.

216 (a) Strawberry cervix.
(b) Trichomonas vaginalis.
(c) It is a unicellular organism with four flagellae and an undulating membrane.
(d) Metronidazole, 200 mg, three times daily, for one week or larger doses over a shorter period. The patient's partner should be treated also.

217 (a) Polycystic ovarian disease. Note the small fimbrial cyst.
(b) Oligomenorrhoea, infertility, obesity and hirsutism.
(c) LH/FSH both increased with a ratio greater than 3:1, the androstenedione and testosterone levels may be elevated.
(d) About half of the patients will have increased vascularity of the breasts which, in conjunction with periods of amenorrhoea, often suggests that the patient might be pregnant when she is not.

218 (a) Testicular feminisation syndrome because of well developed breasts and lack of pubic hair. Testosterone levels will be in the normal range of males and cystogenetic studies will show a 46 XY genotype.
(b) A short vagina, with an absent uterus.
(c) The gonads should be removed because of the risk of malignancy.
(d) There is androgen insensitivity due to absent androgen receptors and, therefore, failed development of external male genitalia and male secondary characteristics. The female phenotype develops by default.

219 (a) No.
(b) From the squamo-columnar junction and at least at 12 o'clock and 6 o'clock.
(c) Yes.
(d) Yes, illumination and magnification of the cervix and assessment after the application of acetic acid prior to the iodine allows biopsies to be taken from the most abnormal areas.

Potatoes
Spring Onions
Onions
Carrots